JUN   2008

618.92 BENAROCH
Benaroch, Roy.
Solving health and
 behavioral problems fr
2008/05/21

W9-CHO-104

SOLVING HEALTH AND BEHAVIORAL PROBLEMS FROM BIRTH THROUGH PRESCHOOL

SOLVING HEALTH AND BEHAVIORAL PROBLEMS FROM BIRTH THROUGH PRESCHOOL

A Parent's Guide

ROY BENAROCH, M.D.

Alameda Free Library
1550 Oak Street
Alameda, CA 94501

The Praeger Series on Contemporary Health and Living
Julie Silver, Series Editor

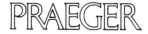

Westport, Connecticut
London

Library of Congress Cataloging-in-Publication Data

Benaroch, Roy.
    Solving health and behavioral problems from birth through preschool : a parent's guide /
Roy Benaroch.
        p.   cm. – (The Praeger series on contemporary health and living, ISSN 1932–8079)
        Includes bibliographical references and index.
        ISBN 978–0–275–99347–4 (alk. paper)
        1. Pediatrics—Popular works.   2. Children—Health and hygiene—Popular works.
3. Children—Diseases—Popular works.   I. Title.
    RJ61.B435   2007
    618.92–dc22   2007023756

British Library Cataloguing in Publication Data is available.

Copyright © 2007 by Roy Benaroch

All rights reserved. No portion of this book may be
reproduced, by any process or technique, without the
express written consent of the publisher.

Library of Congress Catalog Card Number: 2007023756
ISBN-13: 978–0–275–99347–4
ISBN-10: 0–275–99347–7
ISSN: 1932–8079

First published in 2007

Praeger Publishers, 88 Post Road West, Westport, CT 06881
An imprint of Greenwood Publishing Group, Inc.
www.praeger.com

Printed in the United States of America

The paper used in this book complies with the
Permanent Paper Standard issued by the National
Information Standards Organization (Z39.48–1984).

10 9 8 7 6 5 4 3 2 1

This book is for general information only. No book can ever substitute for the judgment of a
medical professional. If you have worries or concerns, contact your doctor.

The names and many details of individuals discussed in this book have been changed to protect the
patients' identities. Some of the stories are composites of patient interactions created for illustrative
purposes.

For Brenda and my Dad

CONTENTS

SERIES FOREWORD

Over the past hundred years, there have been incredible medical break-throughs that have prevented or cured illness in billions of people and helped many more improve their health while living with chronic conditions. A few of the most important twentieth-century discoveries include antibiotics, organ transplants, and vaccines. The twenty-first century has already heralded important new treatments including such things as a vaccine to prevent human papillomavirus from infecting and potentially leading to cervical cancer in women. Polio is on the verge of being eradicated worldwide, making it only the second infectious disease behind smallpox to ever be erased as a human health threat.

In this series, experts from many disciplines share with readers important and updated medical knowledge. All aspects of health are considered including subjects that are disease-specific and preventive medical care. Disseminating this information will help individuals to improve their health as well as researchers to determine where there are gaps in our current knowledge and policymakers to assess the most pressing needs in health care.

Series Editor Julie Silver, M.D.
Assistant Professor
Harvard Medical School
Department of Physical Medicine and Rehabiliation

PREFACE

This book isn't about how doctors solve problems. It's about what parents need to know to fix problems on their own.

The practice of medicine has changed. In the past, the relationship between a physician and patient was mostly a one-way street. Sure, the patient would have a few words to say at first, but it was the doctor who made the important decisions. The exchange was simple and quick, but not in any way informative: "This is what is wrong, and these are the pills you need to take." Real information was kept guarded, only known by true inside medical professionals.

To make the best medical decisions for children, information needs to go in both directions. The doctor needs to know what's going on with the child, but parents also need to know the medical information and science that helps guide the best care. The exchange needs to be two-way, with the doctor acting as a guide and teacher.

In the long run, this sort of doctor-family relationship can not only lead to better medical decisions, but also to more confident and able parents. There's far too much new knowledge developing every day for any single doctor to know everything, and parents can offer new ideas and perspectives. Each child's health history and personality is unique, and parents have a keen ability to understand exactly what symptoms mean in their own individual children. Just sensing when something is really wrong can be a genuine asset in a medical evaluation, and a good doctor should take advantage of parents' special skills in knowing their own kids. By teaching and guiding in a two-way conversation, pediatricians can help parents understand the health and behavioral needs of their children and become less dependent on doctors in the future.

Doctors not only provide information, but also judgment and context and wisdom. We've probably seen your problem many times before, and we've got a feel for what it ought to look like and what's likely to fix it. We've also had the training and experience to have seen the rare stuff—the serious things you hope your child doesn't have. An exceptional doctor teaches parents about their main concern, but also keeps a sensitive eye out for the uncommon things that really need to be addressed right away. Though at least 95 percent of what pediatricians see in our offices isn't serious, having a good two-way relationship with your child's pediatrician will help both of you stay sharp at spotting the other 5 percent.

This book teaches parents the essential facts about behavioral and medical issues that confront families from birth through the preschool years. The most common problems are reviewed, including preventing and treating ordinary infections; evaluating and alleviating symptoms like fever, cough, and ear pain; controlling allergies and asthma; and teaching children to behave. Sleeping and eating skills do not come automatically, and understanding how these abilities develop can help parents overcome struggles and confrontations at mealtimes and bedtime. Parents of newborns will learn about dealing with colic and gas in a way that doesn't require medication, helping baby and parents develop better relationships together.

The information in this book is based on the best current science and evidence, without holding back any secrets. It covers what state-of-the-art medicine should be—even when it might contradict what some doctors are doing. If you're the parent of a baby or young child, what you need to know most about the health and behavior of your child is right here.

No book can replace a family's pediatrician. Though you'll learn the most important facts and inside information about common problems, your own pediatrician's compassion and understanding are going to be necessary for many issues that complicate children's lives. The relationship between doctors and patients has changed, but parents still want to know how to take care of their kids the way a true insider would. The best-informed parents are best at taking care of their kids, and this book will help get you started.

ACKNOWLEDGMENTS

I want to thank the doctors who've inspired me most to listen, to learn, and to think.

Lee Benaroch	Patty de Urioste	Bob Pettignano
Frank Berkowitz	Lorne Garrettson	Charles Sewell
John Boring	David Goo	Joseph Snitzer
Susie Buchter	Robert Gunn	Neill Videlefsky
Jack Burstiner	David Lloyd	W. Dean Wilcox
J. Devn Cornish	Bhagirath Majmudar	

Thanks also to my sweetheart Jodi for her patience, encouragement, and editing skills.

Special thanks to my patients and my own kids for teaching me so much about children. There's *always* more to learn.

1

PREVENTING INFECTIONS: AN OUNCE OF PREVENTION

Preventing disease is *always* better than treating disease. Public health, vaccinations, clean and safe food and water—these and other preventive strategies are the best ways to keep as many children as possible healthy and safe.

In children, many health problems are triggered by infections. The common cold, pink eye, pneumonia, strep throat, and diarrhea are all usually avoidable if you keep your child away from germs. Of course, the germs themselves will not make this easy. They've developed clever ways to spread and reach as many children as possible:

- Pink eye makes eyes itchy and painful. So eyes get rubbed—and guess what's now all over the child's hands? The next doorknob or toy that is touched will have infectious germs on it, and the next person to touch the same object is very likely to end up with the same infection.
- Likewise, the mucus and runny nose that appears in such abundance during a cold is loaded with infectious viruses. This is especially true at the start of the cold, before a child really seems sick. When itchy, watery noses are rubbed, hands become very effective at spreading disease.
- Diarrhea can be loaded with infectious germs, too. And unfortunately it sometimes gets *everywhere*. It's tough to make sure that surfaces exposed to diarrhea are well sanitized. When one kid in diapers has diarrhea, it quickly spreads to every child and adult at day care. From there, other family members become victims.

In the developed world, most of these infections are more of a nuisance than serious—but anyone who's spent the night washing sheets and holding a baby with vomiting and diarrhea would gladly do without the experience! Sometimes minor infections can lead to serious complications. Preventing germs from spreading is a crucial way to keep your child healthy.

HAND WASHING AND HYGIENE

Gloria has seemed to be sick ever since starting day care at eighteen months. She'll get one head cold, then a cough for a while; after just a few clear days she seems to be congested again. Some weeks she has vomiting, and other weeks diarrhea. One illness runs right into the next! Despite this, Gloria seems to like day care. She's growing well and developing normally, and in between illnesses she's her usual happy self.

Almost all ordinary infections—those that cause colds, pink eye, diarrhea, vomiting, strep throat, most pneumonias, and even serious infections like meningitis—are spread through contact with contaminated surfaces. (A few infections can sometimes spread through the air, including chicken pox, measles, and tuberculosis.) Normal toddlers like Gloria spend their time in group care touching everything and everybody in the room, so it should be no surprise that these children get so many infections.

> ☞ **The best way to prevent the transmission of most infections is to keep hands clean.**

The single most effective way to prevent common infections is with frequent and thorough hand washing. Hands should be washed before eating, after touching sick people, and several extra times each day. Health care workers should wash their hands before and after every single patient contact. A good hand washing requires running water, plenty of soap, and vigorous friction (rubbing). It takes about forty-five seconds to thoroughly wash hands. Regular, ordinary soap is fine; antibacterial soap offers no advantage.

Rubbing hands with a hand sanitizer (Purell, and many other brand and generic products) containing about 60 percent alcohol gel is a very effective substitute for hand washing. In studies of diarrheal illness and common colds, it is as effective as hand washing—maybe even more so. It also is easier on the skin than using soap. If there is visible dirt, mucus, blood, or any other human material, hands should be washed traditionally with soap and running water.

Some additional hygiene habits can also help. Children should be taught to cough or sneeze into the crook of their elbow rather than into their own hands. You can also *try* to discourage children from putting their hands in their mouth or rubbing their eyes. That's easier said than done in a typical two-year-old!

AVOIDING SICK PEOPLE

All parents who send their children to school or day care have a duty to protect the other children in the group from illness. Children with fever, diarrhea, or other symptoms of infection should be kept home. If every parent could effectively isolate their sick children from group care, it would decrease the number of sick days for children and parents alike.

Unfortunately, this is another suggestion that is sometimes more easily said than done. In truth, a child coming down with a cold is infectious even before she seems sick, and she may show her first signs of illness while she's already at school! Still, try your best to help your community by keeping your child away from others during infectious illnesses.

NUTRITION AND SUPPLEMENTS

Children who are malnourished—that is, who lack vitamins and minerals in their diet, or who just aren't getting enough food—have weakened immune systems. This is rarely seen in the developed world, where food is plentiful and fortified with extra vitamins.

There is no evidence, though, that "supernutrition" is extra protective. Giving mega-doses of vitamin C will not prevent colds, nor will any other special nutritional supplement. Some herbs have been touted to have infection-fighting properties, but the results of well-designed trials have not been able to confirm that any of these products will really help.

If your child is a picky eater who rarely touches fruits or vegetables, it is a good idea to give him a daily multivitamin. An inexpensive generic product is fine. There is no need to spend your money on special "premium" vitamins or any other specific supplement product.

IMMUNIZATIONS

Along with dependably clean food and water, routine immunizations are the greatest public health triumph of the twentieth century. Many very serious diseases have been nearly eradicated from the developed world, and all of our children are far safer because almost all of them are immune from so many serious diseases. That means that not only are vaccinated children protected, but even the most vulnerable among us—newborns, those with serious immune problems, or those who for whatever reason haven't been immunized—are also protected because they are unlikely to come in contact with anyone with one of these diseases.

Unfortunately, the system isn't perfect. Political struggles have set back the effort to completely eliminate polio in Africa, and a misguided antivaccine movement, mostly in the United States and Great Britain, has convinced enough parents to skip immunizations that individual communities have experienced epidemics of measles and mumps that could have been prevented. Vaccines themselves, like any other medicine, are never 100 percent effective, and sometimes immunity is incomplete.

The good news is that newer vaccines are safer and more effective than ever. Studies looking at millions of vaccine doses have failed to confirm any of the hysteria that has led some families to be unnecessarily fearful of vaccines. We are now able to prevent more and more serious infections, including severe diarrhea in infants and the viral infection that causes cervical cancer in women.

Routine childhood vaccines can protect your child from many serious infections, and every parent should follow the nationally published recommendations for routine immunization. Below is a brief overview of the routine vaccines recommended for preschoolers. For more information about vaccines, including more specific and up-to-date information about current vaccine recommendations, risks, and benefits, please refer to the resources listed at the end of this chapter.

DTaP

The vaccine for diphtheria, tetanus, and pertussis is available in several brand names, including some brands that combine this with other vaccines. Diphtheria causes a severe sore throat with neurologic and cardiac problems. Tetanus, also called "lockjaw," is caused by a bacteria that grows in soil all over the world. In addition to muscle spasms, tetanus causes severe, intractable seizures. Pertussis, or "whooping cough," is the most common of these three illnesses. In part, this is from waning immunity as immunized kids get older. Until recently, there was no booster available to keep adults immune. In babies, especially newborns, pertussis can lead to such severe coughing that a child cannot breathe. Not only should babies be immunized, but parents of newborns should also receive booster immunizations to prevent pertussis from affecting their children.

The modern version of this vaccine is called "acellular," and is more purified than what was used in prior generations. Though the older vaccine did commonly cause fevers and rarely more severe reactions, the modern version is very safe and unlikely to cause any problems.

Hepatitis A

Though the immunization has been available for years, until 2007 hepatitis A vaccination was only recommended for travel or for children living in high-risk areas. Now, routine vaccination is recommended for all children in the United States. The illness itself can be quite mild in children, causing abdominal pain and vomiting. But for parents or the elderly, hepatitis A is far more severe. Hepatitis A is spread by contact with infected people or contaminated food.

Hepatitis B

Hepatitis B infects many adults, and can spread to newborns during or after childbirth. Unfortunately, a baby who contracts hepatitis B is very likely to develop chronic disease, eventually leading to cirrhosis or cancer of the liver. Almost all of these cases can be prevented by routine surveillance for hepatitis B among pregnant women and routine vaccination of newborns.

HIB

HIB stands for "*Haemophilus influenzae* type B." This bacteria, which can be spread from person to person, was once one of the most common causes of several serious infections of preschoolers, including meningitis, blood infections, and infections of the tissues of the throat. Though the name of the bacteria includes the word "influenzae," this vaccine actually has nothing to do with influenza vaccination or "the flu."

Influenza

"The flu" is a serious and sometimes fatal illness, causing fevers and misery in millions of people each winter. Vaccinating kids not only keeps them healthy, but prevents them from spreading disease to their families, schools, and communities. To maintain immunity, influenza vaccination needs to be repeated every winter. Though most children have been vaccinated with a "flu shot," a safe and effective nasal spray flu vaccine may soon be available for preschoolers.

MMR

MMR stands for "measles, mumps, and rubella." In addition to the rash, measles causes severe pneumonia which in the past was often fatal. Mumps causes painful swelling of the neck, and can also include swelling of the brain and other serious complications. Though rubella, also called "German Measles," is a mild illness, if it strikes a pregnant woman the baby will have severe birth defects and brain damage. All of these illnesses have become very rare in the United States, but occasional outbreaks continue to occur, usually traced to individuals who chose to skip vaccination, traveled overseas, and brought these infections back with them.

Pneumococcal Conjugate

By preventing infections caused by the bacteria pneumococcus, this vaccine prevents meningitis, blood infections, and pneumonia. To a lesser degree, it can help prevent at least some ear infections. Routine vaccination with pneumococcal conjugate and HIB vaccines has made bloodstream infections and meningitis quite rare in young children. The pneumococcal conjugate vaccine is usually called by its trade name, "Prevnar."

Polio

The World Health Organization has targeted polio for complete eradication, and at the beginning of this century public heath officials were very close to that goal. However, political strife and deliberate misinformation campaigns have led to a resurgence of polio in the developing world. Sadly, complete eradication of polio may not be attainable. Imported cases of polio are still occurring even in the Western world, so routine vaccination against this very serious illness is still necessary.

Rotavirus

Rotavirus causes most cases of vomiting and diarrhea illnesses in the winter. It's not only a truly miserable experience—severe dehydration from rotavirus also causes several dozen deaths each year among babies in the United States. Rotaviral illness is one of the most common reasons for pediatric emergency room visits and hospitalizations. The rotavirus vaccine is given orally to babies between two and six months.

Varicella

Also called "chicken pox," varicella in most cases is a five-day nuisance of itching, fevers, and missed school. However, some children do have serious complications, leading to approximately fifty deaths each year in the United States. Worse, children with chicken pox can spread disease to older people or other individuals at high risk for complications. Besides protecting the child and contacts from chicken pox, varicella vaccination also protects children from shingles. New recommendations call for a second, "booster" dose of varicella vaccine for all children to prevent mild disease and contagion. With the establishment of this second dose, it will be possible to make chicken pox as rare as measles, or eliminate it completely.

Simple steps are the best ways to prevent infections in your child: wash or sanitize hands, get vaccinated, and avoid sick people. Even with the most careful parents, every child is bound to pick up an infection at least once in a while. If the infection is caused by a bacteria, antibiotic medicines may be an important part of the cure. In the next chapter, we'll look at the pound of cure that might be needed when an ounce of prevention fails.

VACCINE INFORMATION RESOURCES

Vaccine information changes rapidly as new vaccines are developed and new studies are released concerning their safety and effectiveness. The best, most up-to-date information can be found on trustworthy, honest, and complete sites on the Internet. But keep in mind that there is a great deal of misinformation and hysteria about vaccines on the World Wide Web, too. Be especially wary of undocumented claims, unreferenced or undated articles, or information that cannot be easily confirmed through well-established venues. To find reliable, up-to-date, and scientifically valid information, start with one of the Web sites listed below.

http://www.cdc.gov/nip
http://www.vaccineinformation.org
http://www.vaccine.chop.edu

2

TREATING INFECTIONS: A POUND OF CURE

The development of effective treatments for infection has been one of the greatest medical advances in human history. Millions of lives have been improved or saved with the availability of these agents, which can effectively help patients recover from infections that used to be the most common causes of death and misery. In the mid-twentieth century it was believed that modern antibiotics would make infections a thing of the past.

Fifty years has made a big difference. Now, doctors are trying to play catch-up. Our older, safer antibiotics are becoming less effective, and some common bacterial infections are becoming very difficult to treat. New and emerging infections are also testing our ability to quickly come up with new treatments.

Antibiotics have become less effective because they have been used far too much. Indiscriminate use of antibiotics allows bacteria to develop resistance, and resistance among one bacterial type can easily spread to others. Even if your own child has never been on antibiotics, she likely has been exposed to bacteria that have developed resistance while infecting other people. Preventing antibiotic resistance requires more than just keeping your own child off antibiotics. As a society, we must strive to administer antibiotics in the best way: use the correct antibiotic for the correct length of time and only when necessary.

Using antibiotics unnecessarily exposes your child to other risks as well. There are allergic reactions that can be serious or fatal. Less severe adverse effects are common: diarrhea, upset stomach, or vomiting. In a subtle way, overreliance on antibiotics may encourage families to depend too much on their doctors. That is, families who have learned to always expect an antibiotic prescription will begin to feel that they must seek their doctor's advice for every illness, however minor. Once families and doctors start using antibiotics routinely for every ailment, it can be a hard habit to break.

DECISION #1: IS AN ANTIBIOTIC NECESSARY?

Antibiotics, by their nature, only treat bacterial infections. (There are medicines that can treat *some* viral infections. These are called "antivirals" and are covered briefly at the end of this chapter.) They weaken bacterial organisms so that the body's immune system can kill them off. Antibiotics are not meant to be 100 percent effective in killing bacteria alone; they are only given to help a natural immune system fight off infection. In children with impaired immunity for any reason, treating infection is more difficult.

Why Are Antibiotics Overused?

It is no secret that doctors have been quick to prescribe antibiotics for viral infections. I am sad to say that many doctors continue to do this, despite widespread and well-established educational opportunities to keep physicians better informed. Why do doctors prescribe antibiotics that are not needed?

- *Patient satisfaction.* Some doctors believe parents will be disappointed if they do not get a prescription, but studies have shown that parents will be just as happy without a prescription *if* the doctor explains why an antibiotic is unnecessary and takes the time to discuss other ways of helping the child.
- *Speed.* It's true: any doc can more quickly write a prescription than talk about why one isn't needed.
- *Dependence.* Families who begin to depend on an antibiotic prescription for viral infections are more likely to see their doctor for every ailment. Is it possible that some doctors deliberately or subconsciously overprescribe to increase future business and revenue?

Your doctor, after discussing the history and performing a physical exam, will determine the most likely diagnosis, and will know how likely it is that a bacterial infection is present. Sometimes, tests can be used to confirm a bacterial infection, such as a urine culture for a urinary tract infection, or a strep test for bacterial strep throat. Usually, though, you will rely on the experience and skill of the physician to make the diagnosis.

If the diagnosis is a likely bacterial infection, the next question is whether it is likely to get better on its own. For instance, most ear infections will improve without antibiotics, though antibiotics can relieve pain faster and prevent complications. Many factors should be considered before automatically using an antibiotic for a bacterial infection:

- How sick is the child?
- What will likely happen without antibiotics?
- Will the child be able to tell us if she's getting sicker?

- Can the family come back or get in touch with the doctor if there's trouble?
- Is there a safe and effective antibiotic available?
- Do drug allergies complicate the decision?

Because of the serious consequences of antibiotic overuse, we can no longer make an automatic decision based on just the diagnosis. Deciding whether to treat a child with antibiotics requires careful judgment by both the doctor and the parents of a child.

> ☞ **Most infections in children are viral. Antibiotics won't help.**

Is an Antibiotic Necessary for Most Childhood Ailments?

Bronchiolitis	No
Bronchitis	No
Common cold	No
Cough	Rarely
Croup	No
Diarrhea	No
Ear infection	Sometimes
Fever	Antibiotics should not be prescribed for a fever unless a more specific diagnosis is made
Pink eye	No oral antibiotics
Pneumonia	Sometimes
Sinusitis	Sometimes
Sore throat	No, unless it is caused by strep
Strep throat	Yes
Upper respiratory infection	No
Urinary tract infection	Yes
Vomiting	No

Note: For more information about the best way to treat these problems, see their individual chapters or the index.

DECISION #2: HOW TO GIVE IT

Topical antibiotics are creams or drops than can be applied at the site of infection. These can be used for small skin infections, eye infections, infections of the outer ear canal, or middle ear infections in children who have tubes.

By using a topical agent, a high concentration of antibiotic can be put exactly where it needs to go without exposing the rest of the body to the drug. There's far less chance of significant allergy, side effects, or the development of resistance when topical agents are used.

If a topical agent is impractical or cannot reach the site of infection, an oral antibiotic can be prescribed. These can be in liquids, chewables, or pills. Choose the form that your child is most likely to accept. Ask if the liquid tastes reasonably good, and try to choose a medication that can be given less frequently or for fewer days.

There are two commonly used injected antibiotics. These are very useful in a child who is vomiting, or when a more serious infection makes it essential to quickly get a high dose of antibiotic on board. There are disadvantages to injections: allergic reactions can be more severe, and future doctor visits may be more difficult if the child remembers painful shots! Injections should not be used solely for convenience.

DECISION #3: WHICH ANTIBIOTIC?

Dozens of antibiotics are available. Choosing which one to use means looking at several factors:

Spectrum. An antibiotic's spectrum refers to which bacteria it kills effectively. There is no such thing as a "strong" antibiotic; different antibiotics kill different bacteria well. If a certain antibiotic is effective against the bacteria you're trying to treat, consider it "strong." Being able to kill every bacteria on the block doesn't make an antibiotic "stronger," it just makes it more likely to cause side effects and foster antibiotic resistance. Given a choice, it is much better to choose a "narrow-spectrum" antibiotic that kills exactly the bacteria you're trying to get rid of rather than a "broad-spectrum" antibiotic that kills lots of bacteria that aren't harming you. The difference can be compared to a rifle versus a shotgun: choose the narrow-spectrum rifle, which kills exactly what it's aimed at, rather than the shotgun that also ruins the nearby house and furniture. There are times when a more broad-spectrum antibiotic is necessary—especially if many different organisms cause the same infection. But in general, narrow is the way to go. And there's a bonus: narrow-spectrum antibiotics tend to be older, safer, and cheaper.

Tissue penetration. Certain antibiotics get to different places in the body once they're swallowed. Zithromax (azithromycin), for instance, penetrates lung tissue well but isn't a good choice to treat an infection in the urine. Not all antibiotics are suitable to treating infections in all parts of the body.

Price. Someone is paying for the antibiotic—either the patient or the insurance company. And the insurance company will pass along the costs of expensive drugs to whomever is paying the premiums. Though newer antibiotics are marketed very heavily to doctors and sometimes directly to patients, they often offer no advantage over older, less-expensive drugs. Expensive brand name medicines are rarely needed.

Formulary availability. If your insurance covers the cost of drugs, you may need to look in a booklet to know which medicines are covered at the lowest cost. Generics are almost always low-cost, so choose those and you'll be fine.

Dosing forms. Your pediatrician knows which medicines come in pills, liquids, chewables, or other forms. Since young children can't swallow pills, we also know which liquids taste good!

ANTIBIOTICS COMMONLY USED IN CHILDREN

This is not meant to be an exhaustive list, but rather a brief, practical introduction to the antibiotics a pediatrician is likely to prescribe. Information about generic availability is current with the printing of this edition. Because medicines are most commonly called by their most-popular brand names, I've listed those first in most cases throughout this book. Generic and other alternative names appear in parentheses. All of these medications are available as pills or capsules and liquids unless otherwise noted.

Amoxil (amoxicillin) [generic available]. The classic "pink stuff" tastes great to most kids. It's also cheap, and it works well for many childhood infections. It's commonly used for ear infections, sinusitis, and pneumonia; in some parts of the country it remains a good antibiotic for urinary tract infections as well. Though strep bacteria have never learned to be resistant to amoxicillin, over the past few decades there has been a small but steady increase in the proportion of strep throats that don't seem to get better with this medication. Amoxicillin comes in many forms: a tasty liquid, chewables, or surprisingly large pills. It is usually taken twice a day.

Augmentin (amoxicillin/clavulanate) [generic available] adds a second ingredient to amoxicillin to cover some resistant bacteria. It is relatively inexpensive as a generic, tastes okay, and is taken twice a day. It is available in two forms: a traditional strength (called "Augmentin" or "Augmentin 400") and an "extra strength" (called "Augmentin ES" or "Augmentin 600"). The extra strength improves its effectiveness against infections in the chest and upper respiratory tract, including ear infections, sinusitis, and pneumonia—but it does *not* increase its effectiveness in urinary tract infections nor skin infections. As with many antibiotics, it has become less effective against infections in the skin and should not routinely be used for this any more. It comes in a very large pill, liquid, or a chewable.

Bactrim (trimethoprim sulfamethoxazole, also known as Septra or co-trimoxizole) [generic available]. Bactrim is the most widely used of the older group of "sulfa" antibiotics, and has become much more popular again because it has remained effective against most skin infections caused by the resistant staph bacteria called "MRSA." Once seen only in hospitalized patients, MRSA is now common in most communities in the United States, causing skin abscesses, boils, and impetigo. Often, the infections look like an "infected spider bite." MRSA can also cause more serious problems such as pneumonia or bone infections (osteomyelitis.) Only a small number of oral antibiotics appropriate for children remain effective against it, including Bactrim and clindamycin. Unfortunately, with the increased use of Bactrim we will probably soon see that it will lose its power against MRSA. Bactrim is also used for urinary tract infections or as a second-line agent for ear infections or sinusitis—though it is becoming less effective for these, and should probably be reserved for its unique power against skin infections. The liquid form of Bactrim tastes okay and is taken twice a day. Unfortunately, Bactrim can rarely trigger a very serious skin allergy. If your child develops a rash, red lips, or red eyes while on Bactrim stop the medication and call your doctor.

Cleocin (clindamycin) [generic available]. Traditionally known by its generic name, clindamycin is most useful for skin infections, including MRSA. It's also suitable as second-line therapy for strep throat, ear infections, and sinusitis. Clindamycin does not enjoy much popularity because of the terrible taste of its liquid form. If it has to be used, go with the capsule form and sprinkle or crush it for children who can't swallow it whole. It should be given three or more times a day, and can cause diarrhea.

Keflex (cephalexin) [generic available]. Keflex is one of the first of a group of "cephalosporin" antibiotics. It has excellent effectiveness against strep throat, and depending on the area of the country it may be the drug of choice for urinary tract infections. Because of the rapid spread of resistant staph bacteria, Keflex is no longer a good choice for skin infections. Keflex is cheap, tastes good, and is usually taken two or three times a day. *Duricef (cefadroxil)* [generic available] is not used as widely but is quite similar to Keflex.

Omnicef (cefdinir) [no generic available]. Omnicef is the most popular of the newer cephalosporin antibiotics, though it is expensive. It's heavily promoted for ear and sinus infections, and may be a good second choice if amoxicillin fails because it does provide more "broad" coverage. It's also used for skin infections, though it is ineffective against resistant staph bacteria. Omnicef has a pleasant taste, and can be taken once a day. Occasionally, children taking Omnicef develop red stools that can look like blood. Two similar drugs, *Ceftin (cefuroxime)* [generic available as pill only] and *Vantin (cefpodoxime)* [no generic available], are used less frequently than Omnicef because of the unpleasant taste of their liquid forms. Other related medicines in this group, including *Cedax (ceftibuten), Lorabid (loracarbef)* [no generics available], and *Cefzil (cefprozil)* [generic available], should not be first choices for most pediatric infections.

Penicillin [generic available] was one of the first antibiotics, and remains very effective for strep throat and other infections involving the mouth, teeth, and gums. Its liquid form is bitter, so pediatricians often prescribe its cousin amoxicillin for children who can't swallow pills. For most infections, penicillin is given two to four times a day. Penicillin can be given by injection, usually in cases of strep throat accompanied by vomiting. Penicillin injections are big and thick and hurt far more than a vaccine. They can rarely lead to a very serious allergic reaction. Penicillin injections should never be a first choice.

Rocephin (ceftriaxone) [for injection only]. This is a very effective agent for many serious and not-too-serious infections of childhood, from simple ear infections to meningitis, pneumonia, and bloodstream infections. It should be reserved for children who are ill and either can't tolerate or haven't responded to oral medications. Because it is such an important tool in offices and emergency rooms, Rocephin should only be used when necessary. As with other antibiotics, overuse will lead to bacterial resistance and decreasing effectiveness.

Suprax (cefixime) [generic available, but it is often still expensive] is an excellent, good tasting, once-a-day medication for urinary tract infections, though it is more expensive than Keflex. It has few other uses.

Zithromax (azithromycin) [generic available]. Zithromax has some unique advantages. It can be taken only once a day for only one to five days, and tastes reasonably okay. When it was first introduced, it was a good choice for common infections like strep throat and ear infections. However, the popularity of Zithromax became its undoing: it is no longer very effective against most childhood infections. Many strep germs and common ear infection triggers are resistant, and Zithromax has limited usefulness for sinus infections or skin infections. It's still a reasonable second-line medication to try in children who are allergic to other agents. The waning usefulness of Zithromax is a good example of how antibiotic overuse can quickly help bacteria become resistant. *Biaxin (clarithromycin)* [no generic available] and *erythromycin* [generic available] have similar spectrums of activity, and have similarly lost their punch for

> ☞ **Which antibiotic is best depends on what infection is being treated and many other factors. Though some antibiotics are better than others for an individual case, no antibiotic is "stronger" than any other for every infection.**

most childhood infections. Because of the poor taste of its liquid form and requirement for twice-a-day dosing, Biaxin never became quite as popular as Zithromax in pediatrics. Erythromycin has the additional disadvantages of three- or four-times-a-day dosing and more frequent gastrointestinal (GI) side effects.

USING ANTIBIOTICS WISELY

To get the best results in the safest manner, follow these tips:

- Measure doses carefully, and complete the entire prescription as ordered.
- Do not save leftovers or hoard antibiotics for later use.
- Store the medication as indicated on the label. Accidentally leaving a "must be refrigerated" antibiotic out for a few hours or overnight at room temperature will not decrease its effectiveness, but leaving it in a hot car will. If you're in doubt about storage, contact your pharmacist.
- If you're late for a dose, make it up as soon as possible; if you've skipped one or two doses entirely, just continue at the prescribed amount when you remember. If you've missed more than a few doses, contact your physician for instructions.
- If your child "spits up" a dose within fifteen minutes, repeat it. If this happens more than once, contact your doctor.

• Read the label for instructions regarding whether to take the medication with or without food.

What to Do about Side Effects

Contact your physician if side effects occur, including vomiting, diarrhea, or rashes. You'll need to get more specific instructions from your own physician who knows the overall picture well. She may suggest holding a dose, reducing the dose, changing the antibiotic, or treating the side effects symptomatically.

If a significant side effect or adverse reaction occurs, you or your doctor's office should report this to the Food and Drug Administration's Medwatch program via http://www.fda.gov/medwatch/.

Other Uses of Antibiotics

Antibiotics are usually prescribed to treat known or suspected bacterial infections. There are some other uses:

"Back-up." Sometimes called a "Safety Net Antibiotic Prescription," some practitioners will encourage symptomatic treatment of some common infections, giving an antibiotic prescription only to be used as a backup if the child worsens. This strategy can reduce the overall use of antibiotics, while allowing parents to feel more in control and able to respond should their child have trouble. If your doctor uses this approach, make sure you understand exactly how to decide if you need to fill the prescription. If you do fill the prescription, use the complete course. Do not hoard an unused prescription for next time.

Foreign travel. Antibiotics should be brought with a family for travel to certain areas, especially when there is a high risk of diarrheal illness in an area with poor access to health care. Work with your doctor to decide if this is appropriate for your family. More information is available at http://www.cdc.gov/travel/.

Infectious contacts. In a few specific cases, persons in contact with patients who have certain serious or difficult-to-control infections should receive antibiotics. This includes close contacts of people with pertussis (whooping cough) or some kinds of bacterial meningitis. In most cases, though, the best prevention is with hand washing and avoidance of contact rather than antibiotics. There is no need for healthy people in contact with common infections such as pink eye, strep throat, or pneumonia to receive preventative antibiotics.

Prevention, or prophylaxis. Continuous, daily antibiotic administration can be used carefully, in selected high-risk patients, to prevent certain infections of the urinary tract, ears, or other areas. This approach should be used with caution, and may in fact lead to more problems with resistant bacteria.

What to Do if an Antibiotic Doesn't Work

Lyla was brought to a physician after three days of sore throat followed by nasal congestion. Though no strep test was performed, the doctor was "sure it was strep" and started the child on Zithromax. After three days, her symptoms have persisted.

Antibiotics, like other medicines, do not always work. There are several possible reasons:

- The diagnosis could be wrong—that is, perhaps your child has a viral infection after all. Many infections are diagnosed clinically. This means that your doctor's overall impression guides therapy, without confirmation by any sort of test. A common example of this would be antibiotics prescribed for sinus infections. As explained in more detail in Chapter 8, it can be difficult to tell a true bacterial sinus infection from a long viral cold. Many times when antibiotics don't work for a sinus infection it is because in truth the infection is caused by a virus. Changing antibiotics in this case will not help. In Lyla's case, she doesn't have a bacterial infection at all. Her symptoms are much more typical of a common cold, and no antibiotic will help.
- The medication isn't being used right. Sometimes a doctor's writing is tough for the pharmacist to decipher, and patients end up with a wrong drug or wrong dose. Double check with your physician by reading back the bottle, and also be sure to know the dosing instructions for all medicines before you leave your doctor's office.
- There may be unrealistic expectations. It takes time for antibiotics to help your body overcome an infection. It may take two to three days before your child feels well on an antibiotic, even when it's working.
- The antibiotic may be ineffective against the infection. Antibiotic resistance is a common problem seen in the treatment of almost every childhood infection, from simple skin infections to sinusitis to urinary tract infections and pneumonia. Your pediatrician should keep an eye on resistance patterns in your community to help choose the antibiotic that's most likely to work.

Get the information you need before you start the antibiotic—what is it, what's the dose, and how soon should there be improvement? When should you call if the child isn't getting better? Don't assume that you'll always need a new, "stronger" antibiotic, though sometimes it is necessary to change medicines to overcome a resistant bug. Call your doctor if you feel your child isn't getting better as expected.

ANTIVIRAL MEDICINES

Most common viral infections, including those that cause coughs, colds, vomiting, and diarrhea, cannot be fought with medications. However, some antivirals have been developed for specific infections. In general, antivirals are somewhat less effective than antibiotics. Though they help the immune system fight infection, the response to antivirals is not as dramatic, complete, or as quick as the expected response to an antibiotic. Also, most antivirals must be started within the first day or so of a viral infection to have any impact whatsoever. Some of the common viral infections for which antiviral therapy is helpful are:

- *Chicken pox.* If started early on, antiviral medicine can shorten the course of chicken pox or make it milder. This is especially useful in people with immune problems or the very young.
- *Cold sores.* Again, they have to be started quickly, but antiviral medicines fight cold sores caused by herpes simplex virus.
- *HIV.* There are a large number of anti-HIV medicines available; if your child has been exposed to HIV or has HIV infection you should be working with a specialist well versed in recent advances in this developing field.
- *Influenza.* A few different medicines are available to either help treat a proven influenza infection or help prevent its spread to family members. Better yet, rely on vaccination to protect your family.

FOR MORE INFORMATION

http://www.cdc.gov/getsmart. This site, sponsored by the United States Government Centers for Disease Control, has an extensive collection of well-referenced articles for patients, families, and health care workers about the best ways to use antibiotics.

3

FEVER

Almost all of the serious illnesses that caused fever in the past are now rare in the developed world, thanks to vaccinations and improved public health. Measles, blood poisoning (or "sepsis"), polio, and most causes of meningitis are now prevented by routine immunizations, and have become very rare. Infections that still do occur can be effectively treated. Our ability to prevent, diagnose, and treat almost all serious causes of fever means that parents today do not have to worry nearly as much as our grandparents did.

Nonetheless, a fever will make your child feel miserable. Children with fevers can have headaches, glassy eyes, and a rapid pulse. They can sometimes act alarmingly ill, especially when a fever gets over 102°F. Fortunately, fever in a preschooler can usually be safely treated at home. Parents just need to know the inside tips: how to manage a fever, and when the pediatrician really does need to be called.

Fever in a Newborn

The chapter focuses on fevers in otherwise healthy children from age three months to school age. If your baby is less than three months old and feels warm or acts ill, measure the temperature with a rectal thermometer. If the measurement is greater than 100.4°F, call your pediatrician right away. Babies of this age may rapidly become seriously ill with infections, and do not have adequate protection from their own immunity or from vaccines. For these young babies, don't hesitate to call your doctor immediately for any measured fever.

WHAT IS A FEVER?

A fever is a body temperature elevated above normal. Just what number constitutes a fever is not uniformly agreed on even by pediatricians, but most of us consider anything measured above 100.4°F or 100.8°F to be abnormal. The "best," or most standardized, way of measuring a temperature is rectally, but there is no reason to put children through that procedure once they're older than three months. For most preschool-age children, a thermometer held under the armpit (the "axillary" temperature) will give a reading that's accurate enough. Another good, reliable way of measuring temperature is a temporal artery thermometer. These look like a blunt, skinny sort of hammer. You gently sweep the device across a child's forehead to instantly measure the temperature.

To communicate clearly with your pediatrician, say the number that was measured and the method it was done: "It was 102.3, measured with an axillary thermometer." Don't add a degree, as that just confuses people. There is no direct comparison between axillary, rectal, and forehead temperatures, so this business of adding degrees can be misleading. Worse, it may make you think that your child's normal temperature, say 99.6°F, is in fact abnormal if you add a degree and get to 100.6°F. Use your thermometer correctly and consistently, and record the number that it displays.

Your own touch is an excellent screening tool for fever in your own children. Feel a forehead or a tummy, and you'll probably know if your child's temperature is high. However, we do a poor job of estimating the exact temperature with our touch. In other words: if your child doesn't feel warm, you don't need to use a thermometer. But if your child does feel feverish, measure his temperature with a thermometer to help monitor how he's doing.

IS THE FEVER SERIOUS?

Almost all fevers in children are caused by infections. Most commonly, the infections are triggered by viruses that run their course within a few days. In general, the height of a fever correlates with how serious the infection is likely to be. That is, a temperature higher than 104°F is somewhat more likely to be caused by a serious viral or bacterial infection than a lower temperature. However, there are too many exceptions to this for the height of fever to be a reliable indicator. Appendicitis is an example of a serious problem that often occurs with only a low-grade fever; while the innocuous virus that causes roseola can trigger a fever of 105°F! Some practitioners feel that a fever's response to therapy also predicts how serious the underlying problem is—if this were true, you would worry more about a fever that didn't decrease after Tylenol. But this is also an inexact and potentially misleading way to look at fevers.

The best way to know if a fever is caused by a serious problem is to pay close attention to how your child feels *after* you've treated the fever. Children feel miserable and look terrible when their temperature is high, so try to put off deciding whether to make that trip to the emergency room until after the fever medicine has kicked in. Once the fever starts to come down you can better judge how likely your child is to need urgent medical attention. If you are very worried that your child is acting ill, give a dose of fever reducer on your way to the doctor. You and the doctor will both be better able to judge the severity of illness after the medicine is working.

> *Case #1.* Audrey is eighteen months old. She is running a fever of 103°F, and feels miserable. She's crying and whiney, and can't get comfortable. A half-hour after taking Advil, her temperature is down to 101°F. She is reading a book in mom's lap. She's not quite her-self, but is smiling a little bit and interactive. She clearly feels much better.

> *Case #2.* Nearly identical story, but eighteen-month old Kenny's tem-perature came down to 99.5°F after ibuprofen. Unfortunately, he still feels miserable. He's listless, lying down, and staring; when his parents try to console him, he cries and cries.

I am worried about Kenny in Case #2. Although his fever came down, he's *acting* sick. He should be evaluated for his fever, now. Though Audrey is clearly not 100 per-cent well, she feels better after her fever reducer medicine. Her evaluation could safely wait a day or so.

> ☞ **The best way to judge if a fever needs urgent evaluation is to see how the child acts once the fever comes down. Treat the fever, then decide.**

WHO NEEDS TO SEE THE DOCTOR?

All babies less than three months of age and any older children who act ill after their fevers are treated should be evaluated quickly. Depending on other circumstances, fevers can sometimes have a "sooner" evaluation (within twelve to twenty-four hours) or a "later" evaluation (a few days). The table below is meant as a general guideline; call your pediatrician for more precise advice.

Evaluate fever now

- Less than three months of age (Do not wait to see how a baby this young responds to treatment. Call your doctor for any fever)
- Acts ill after treatment
- Difficulty breathing

- Has a poor immune system (Sickle Cell Anemia, immune deficiencies, cancer therapy, or not immunized)

Evaluate fever sooner

- Fever > 103°F
- Specific symptoms such as sore throat, ear pain, pain with urination, or a bad cough
- Difficulty doing normal things like walking, talking, or eating and drinking

Evaluate fever later

- Any fever lasting over five days
- Fevers associated with mild rashes. Mild rashes are any rash that goes away with Benadryl, or any rash that blanches—disappears—when you gently stretch the skin

TREATING FEVER

Treat any temperature that is making your child uncomfortable. That is, even if the measured temperature is 99.8°F—not technically a fever—offer treatment if your child is uncomfortable. The opposite of this statement is also true. If a child has a fever but really is acting fine, there's no reason to begin any therapy.

Some practitioners suggest delaying therapy for fever, thinking that fever itself is a valuable tool the body uses to fight infection. Although it is true that under laboratory situations some infections spread more slowly when heated, it is also true that your own immune system doesn't work as well during a fever. There are no studies that show delaying therapy for fevers is likely to help in any important way. If your child feels ill, help her feel better by reducing the fever.

There are only two medicines commonly used to treat fever:

Acetaminophen (Tylenol, generics) can be used at all ages. It effectively reduces fever for about four hours. In cases of large overdoses or in children with preexisting liver disease, acetaminophen can be toxic. In usual doses it is very safe. A suppository of acetaminophen is available (brand name Feverall), but the dose on the package is wrong. More recent research has shown that acetaminophen is not absorbed well rectally, and a different dose should be given. Ask your pediatrician for the correct dosing of rectal acetaminophen.

Ibuprofen (Advil, Motrin, or generics) is approved for use for ages six months and up. It reduces fever for a little longer than acetaminophen, about six hours. Although in usual doses it is safe, prolonged use can cause stomach and kidney problems, especially in children who are dehydrated.

Both of these medicines are safe and effective. I typically recommend generic ibuprofen for children older than six months because of its longer duration, but if you've found that acetaminophen works better in your children, stick with that.

Should parents alternate ibuprofen and acetaminophen to treat fever? I am leery of this strategy. There may be increased adverse reactions, especially if two exhausted parents are trading off drug administration duties and lose track of which medicine is supposed to go next. Giving medicine every three hours can be exhausting! If your child is uncomfortable with fever and it is too early to give the next dose of ibuprofen, it's fine to use a "pinch hitter" dose of acetaminophen. But watch those doses carefully.

Children with fever should be encouraged to drink more fluids. When children run a fever they lose more body water through evaporation, and if they become dehydrated their fevers will worsen. Offer extra fluids appropriate to your child's age. Newborns should nurse more often, and older kids can be offered Popsicles and ice cream. Milk *can* be given to children with fever. Despite what you may have heard, it won't curdle at any human temperature. You can also try a lukewarm water bath or apply cool washcloths to help reduce fever, but never use alcohol.

Remember: the purpose of treating fever is to help children feel better. Treatment does not make the underlying problem go away, and does not prevent any potential complications. Treatment should help the fever go down, but the fever may not go away completely.

A fever can make your child miserable, and can be frightening for parents. Your first job is to help your child feel better by offering hugs, fluids, and fever-reducing medicine. If your child is older than three months and perks up, you can wait to see how the next day goes before deciding whether a trip to the doctor is needed. Review the tips in this chapter so you can keep cool when your child has a fever.

4

SORE THROAT

Only a few different things cause sore throat in young kids. They're usually part of viral infections that are best managed without prescriptions. Less commonly, a sore throat in a child has a bacterial cause that needs antibiotics. With some insider information, parents can manage most sore throats at home, helping their child feel better and preventing the illness from spreading to the rest of the family.

CAUSES AND SYMPTOMS

Almost all sore throats in children less than three years old are triggered by viral illnesses. Typical symptoms include a sore throat plus mild fever for a few days, followed by a head cold with nasal drip, congestion, and cough. The youngest kids might not say their throat hurts, but they'll act fussy and may refuse solid foods.

Strep throat is an infection caused by bacteria named *Streptococcus pyogenes* or "Group A Strep." It doesn't develop from an ordinary viral sore throat. In children older than three, strep throat accounts for about 10 percent of sore throat illnesses. Strep throat begins suddenly, with a fever and throat pain. Viral symptoms like cough, runny nose, and diarrhea are usually absent. Some children with strep throat complain of headaches, abdominal pain, or vomiting. Though strep throats will go away if left untreated, it is important to treat strep throat with antibiotics to limit its spread and prevent rare complications.

RELATED WORDS: TONSILLITIS, PHARYNGITIS

"Pharyngitis" means swelling and redness of the back of the throat, and is the same as a sore throat. "Tonsillitis" refers to swelling and redness of the tonsils, which are little fleshy knobs poking out from the sides at the back of the throat. Tonsillitis can be either viral or bacterial, and should be evaluated and treated exactly the same way as any other sore throat. You may run across a physician who uses the term tonsillitis to mean "a sore throat I want to treat with antibiotics without doing a proper evaluation." Don't accept antibiotics for pharyngitis or tonsillitis unless your physician has proven a bacterial strep infection is present.

PREVENTION

Hand washing or using an alcohol-based hand sanitizer is the best way to prevent the spread of common infections, including strep throat and viral sore throats. Viruses can be sneaky—they're often most contagious the day before symptoms become obvious. To really reduce the spread of these infections, families need to wash hands frequently throughout the winter, not just when someone has a cold.

Children with strep throat should be excluded from group play and school until they feel well and are no longer contagious, usually twenty-four hours after the first dose of antibiotics.

It is not necessary to discard toothbrushes or other household items following an episode of strep throat. Neither the family pet nor family members without symptoms should be tested for strep. It is also unnecessary to retest children who have had strep unless they continue to have symptoms of a strep infection.

DIAGNOSIS

Before you consider taking a child with a sore throat to the doctor, consider whether strep throat is likely. Review the following table to help decide if your child is likely to have strep:

Findings that do *not* suggest strep throat:
- Normal temperature
- Runny nose
- Cough
- Diarrhea

Findings that *could* suggest strep throat:
- Fever
- Sudden onset
- Deep red throat with pus or red stipples on the tonsils
- Large and tender lymph nodes ("glands") in the neck

If your child doesn't have symptoms or findings that suggest strep and is not otherwise very ill, don't rush to the doctor. If you do visit your pediatrician, I would not suggest a strep test be done. In this circumstance, a positive strep test is more likely to mean that the test is wrong than that your child really has a strep throat.

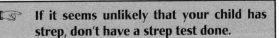 **If it seems unlikely that your child has strep, don't have a strep test done.**

With a careful history and physical examination, even very experienced doctors are only able to correctly determine whether a sore throat is caused by strep about half of the time. That's why every child should have a reliable test performed before starting antibiotics for strep throat.

The standard test for strep throat is a throat culture. However, federal laboratory guidelines prevent many physicians' offices from performing these sorts of tests, which do require some expertise. Most offices now rely on "rapid strep tests," which are more foolproof and take only a few minutes. The best current rapid tests are as good or better than throat cultures because they're easier to perform correctly.

TREATMENT

First, treat the symptoms. Ice cream, milkshakes, and popsicles are as effective as any medicine. Lollipops can help, too. Preschoolers usually don't like throat drops or throat anesthetic sprays like Chloraseptic, though those can help kids willing to try them. You can also try acetaminophen or ibuprofen. These medicines are better at preventing pain than at treating pain. If you know your child's throat is sore, you can get better relief by using these medicines regularly rather than waiting for Junior to complain.

Only proven strep throats should be treated with antibiotics. Occasionally it might make sense to treat a second family member who is getting strep symptoms the day after a sibling had proven strep; there may also be rare times when the physical exam is so suggestive of strep that a negative test might be assumed to be incorrect. But in general, you should insist that your child *not* be given antibiotics unless strep has been proven.

> ☞ **Only sore throats proven to be caused by strep should be treated with antibiotics. Most sore throats are viral, and do not benefit at all from antibiotic therapy.**

There are many antibiotics that can be used to treat strep. Fortunately, the cheapest ones work best. Classic penicillin works well but tastes terrible in liquid form, so most pediatricians substitute tasty amoxicillin. Injectable penicillin works a single dose, but the shot is large and painful. An injection does not work any faster or surer than oral antibiotics taken as directed, but is very useful if your child can't keep oral medicine down. Cephalexin (Keflex) is another older antibiotic that is very effective for strep. For more details about antibiotics that are commonly used in children, see Chapter 2.

> ☞ **Strep throat is best treated with inexpensive, older, and safer antibiotics.**

In all cases, the antibiotic should be taken for the entire course to prevent recurrences, complications, and further doctor visits.

RECURRING STREP

Max was diagnosed with strep throat in early January. He seemed to improve when given his prescribed amoxicillin, one teaspoon once a day. Now, two weeks later, he returns to his pediatrician with a sore throat and fever. Again his strep test is positive.

Some children have a recurrence of strep within a short six-week period. It can be difficult to tell if they've just been unlucky enough to be reexposed, or if their infection has managed to elude antibiotic therapy. If a child has a recurrence of strep, the following steps are the most reasonable:

1. Make sure it really is strep. A child who doesn't have strep symptoms, but tests positive for strep, does not have strep throat and will not benefit from antibiotics. See the next section, "The Strep Carrier."
2. Ensure that antibiotics have been taken as prescribed, for the complete course. In Max's case, his parents misunderstood the directions. They were supposed to have given his medicine twice a day.
3. If penicillin or amoxicillin has been used, try changing to Keflex.
4. If Keflex has been used, treat a recurrence of strep with a combination of two different antibiotics. Often, one of these is rifampin, a unique antibiotic that is able to concentrate in the saliva to coat the tonsils and throat.
5. If three or more proven streps occur in one season, or five or more occur in one year, visit with an ENT surgeon to discuss whether surgery to remove the tonsils is appropriate.

THE STREP CARRIER

This subject deserves special attention, because many physicians are getting this wrong. With your inside information, you may well know how to handle a carrier better than your doctor!

Strep carriers have the strep germ in their throats, yet are not sick. They have no symptoms, and do not spread the infection to anyone else. If given a course of antibiotics, most carriers will briefly lose their strep carriage, but within a few weeks or months they will once again start carrying the bacteria.

Because carriers are not ill and do not spread disease, there is no reason to identify or treat a strep carrier. There is no reason to do strep tests on people who do not have strep symptoms.

> **Do not do strep tests on people who do not have symptoms of strep. You might get a positive result from a carrier, which will only lead to anxiety, worry, and unnecessary antibiotics.**

TONSILLECTOMY

In the past, tonsils were removed for any reason whatsoever—just for looking big, or for vague concerns of speech or swallowing patterns. We now know that even large tonsils seldom do any harm, and there is rarely any need to remove them.

Tonsil tissues themselves are made of infection-fighting cells. They may swell during any sort of infection, viral or bacterial. Though tonsils can be quite large in children, they begin to shrink naturally by age eight. Tonsils should be barely noticeable in most adults.

There are two common reasons to seriously consider surgical removal of tonsils:

1. Recurring strep, with more than three proven strep infections per season or more than five per year. Removal of tonsils reduces the frequency of strep throat by about 90 percent in people who have had frequent strep throat infections.
2. Obstructive sleep apnea, where large tonsils and other throat tissues fold into the airway during sleep, preventing normal breathing. If your child has a loud snore with pauses or gasping breaths, you should speak with your pediatrician about an evaluation for sleep apnea.

A reason NOT to remove tonsils is recurrent nonstrep sore throats. In these kids, the frequent viral infections continue even after tonsillectomy. There's no benefit to undergoing surgery.

SORE THROAT: WHEN TO CALL

> ! These red flags mean call your doctor now:
> - Your child cannot drink.
> - Your child seems especially ill, uncomfortable, or scared.

Contact your pediatrician during regular hours if:

- A sore throat isn't improving after seven days.
- Sore throat is accompanied by a fever over 102°F.
- Your child has recurring strep throats.

Sore throats are common, and can make your child feel bad. Treat the symptoms with love, cool beverages, and pain relievers. Seek a pediatrician's evaluation if your child is miserable or has symptoms that indicate strep throat. Armed with these insider tips, you should be able to make the best decisions for managing your child's next sore throat.

5

EAR INFECTIONS

Acute otitis media, or the common ear infection, is the most commonly encountered bacterial infection in pediatrics. Almost every parent has helped a child struggle through at least one of these painful episodes. Because many children have recurrent ear infections that are difficult to treat, the insertion of ear tubes is the most common surgical procedure performed in the United States (except circumcision.) Unfortunately, many physicians are not consistently taking care of ear infections in the best way. As a parent, understanding the diagnosis and treatment options of ear infections can help you protect your child from unnecessary worry and expensive medications.

> Eighteen-month old Shelly developed a cold the night her mom left on a business trip. Dad's holding down the fort well enough, but on the third night of mom's absence Shelly is in worse shape. She's got a new fever, and she spends the night screaming.

An ear infection means there is infected fluid behind the eardrum. Most, but not all, ear infections are triggered by bacteria that are often found innocently waiting in the upper respiratory tract. These bacteria take advantage of conditions that arise when a child has a common cold—that is, when warm mucus is unable to drain properly from the middle ear. If your child has had a cold for a few days and then gets worsening symptoms such as a new fever, irritability, and wakeful nights, it is likely that the cold has developed into an ear infection. Although most ear infections occur in infants and toddlers, they can affect older children and even adults.

PREVENTION

The best way to prevent an ear infection is to avoid catching a cold: wash or sanitize hands frequently, avoid sick people, and avoid group child care if possible. Breast feeding and some vaccines are also protective. Ear infections are more frequently seen in children exposed to second-hand smoke and in babies fed with a bottle propped upright.

Other strategies to prevent ear infections have been tried, and do not work. Neither cold medicines (decongestants and antihistamines) nor antibiotics help prevent ear infections. Likewise, there is no evidence that any alternative or complementary therapies that are touted to fight colds actually prevent ear infections.

Ear infections have nothing to do with water splashed in the ears. The eardrum is a strong membrane that prevents water or anything else from getting to the middle ear. An ear infection is *behind* the eardrum, not in front of it. In children who have had ear tubes, the surgical opening through the eardrum will allow material to pass though, but that doesn't apply to children who have never had this surgery.

I often distract kids while looking in their ears by talking about the monkeys I see in there. When I started out, I'd just mention the monkeys, but over the years the monkeys have gotten more and more busy. My patients have grown to expect elaborate stories about what the monkeys are doing! One day I walked in an exam room to see a sad five-year-old boy clutching his ear. He told me he had an ear infection "because those monkeys left their banana peels in there!"

DIAGNOSIS

To diagnose an ear infection, your doctor should first ask about how the symptoms developed. The child will usually have had several days of congestion, followed by the sudden onset of ear pain, fussiness, or sleeplessness. A careful physical exam is always required to confirm the diagnosis. The examiner has to prove that there is fluid behind the middle ear, either by seeing outward bulging of the eardrum or by confirming that the eardrum doesn't move when air is blown into the ear canal.

To properly diagnose an ear infection, the examiner has to confirm that there are symptoms of an ear infection *and* fluid behind the eardrum. For the unusual child who really doesn't have symptoms, fluid behind the eardrum is only considered infected if it is bright red. Yellow or cloudy white fluid behind the eardrum of a child who is feeling fine is *not* an ear infection.

Proving that there is both fluid and infection is essential to knowing that a child really has an ear infection. Unfortunately, many physicians seem to get this wrong by either treating yellowish fluid that has no accompanying symptoms, or treating a reddish eardrum that has no fluid behind it. In fact, one reason why antibiotics "don't work"

> ☞ **Don't treat fluid behind the middle ear with antibiotics unless the doctor is sure the fluid is infected. Infected fluid causes fussy symptoms or is bright red.**

is that the child doesn't have an ear infection in the first place. Antibiotics can help with an infection, but they really won't make any difference to an uninfected ear!

Some pitfalls can make the diagnosis of an ear infection especially difficult. Some kids don't appreciate the idea of a warm light in their ear, and fight back. Wax in the ear canal might have to be pulled out, which can lead to an even more upset child who won't hold still. In the same way that crying can make cheeks flush, crying can also make an otherwise normal eardrum bright red. I often hand the otoscope over to a curious child so he can look in my ears first—anything to keep the patient happy! Some tips can help your pediatrician: practice "looking" in your child's ears at home with a toy otoscope, and try to keep wax at bay by gently cleaning the outside of ears with soapy water each day. Please don't use cotton swabs in the ear canal—in a child, that just pushes the wax back farther.

TREATMENT

After a careful exam confirms an ear infection, the most important aspect of treatment is pain control. Pain relief can include a warm compress, an oral medicine such as acetaminophen (Tylenol) or ibuprofen (Motrin, Advil), or numbing eardrops (these work better in children older than five.) Because pain medicines are better at preventing pain than treating pain, once you know your child has an ear infection it is usually best to continue pain medicines around the clock for about twenty-four hours, rather than wait for the child to complain. This is especially true for younger children who can't tell a parent about worsening pain.

Swimmer's Ear

Though not as common as middle ear infections in young children, an infection of the outer ear canal can also cause ear pain. Called "swimmer's ear" or otitis externa, these infections begin when water or other material is trapped in the ear canal, causing the tissues outside of the eardrum to get raw and red. Swimmer's ear can be just as painful as an ordinary ear infection, and the only reliable way to determine which one of these is the culprit is by looking in the ear. Otitis media can be treated with oral antibiotics, but *not* with eardrops; otitis externa should almost always be treated with eardrops.

At least two-thirds of ear infections will resolve on their own, without any antibiotics. But antibiotics can help your child feel better more quickly, and make it more likely that the ear infection will resolve. For children older than two who can clearly communicate symptoms and have had no history of prolonged or recurrent ear infections, a mild infection without much pain can safely be watched for a few days. Antibiotics should be used in children less than two, a child with a fever over 102°F, or any child who is very uncomfortable. Antibiotics should also be used in any child who initially was treated without antibiotics but hasn't improved in a few days.

Which antibiotic treats ear infections best? Though dozens of studies have been done, no antibiotic has ever been shown to be consistently more effective than amoxicillin at the current recommended dose. The newer antibiotics are more likely to lead to diarrhea, stomach upset, and antibiotic resistance. Amoxicillin is cheap, tasty, and can be taken twice a day. It is the best first-line drug for almost everyone, hands down. Other antibiotics should be used when amoxicillin fails or if the patient is allergic. More details about specific antibiotics used in pediatrics are found in Chapter 2.

As is the case with the prevention of ear infections, there is also no evidence that decongestants or other "cold remedies" help treat an ear infection. You might consider these sorts of products if your child is bothered by congestion, cough, or other symptoms of a cold—but they won't help the ear infection heal any faster.

FREQUENT EAR INFECTIONS

What if your child has very frequent ear infections, or ear infections that are difficult to treat? First, try the prevention strategies mentioned above. Be sure you're taking the antibiotic in the best way—consistently and completely. If your child is having recurrent or continuous symptoms despite these measures, the next step would be surgical insertion of ear tubes. (These are more formally called tympanostomy tubes, pressure equalization tubes, or PETs.) The tubes are inserted through the eardrum to drain infected fluid out into the ear canal. Once the fluid can drain, your child should have fewer ear infections. Those that still occur will be far easier and safer to treat by using eardrops rather than oral antibiotics. The tubes are designed to stay in place for about a year. If tubes have been suggested for your child, discuss their risks and benefits both with your pediatrician and with the surgeon who'll be performing the procedure.

Who Needs Tubes for Frequent Ear Infections?

How many ear infections are too many? There's no exact answer. Many factors would push me to encourage the placement of surgical tubes sooner rather than later, as in these children:

- Charlie always requires multiple courses of antibiotics to clear an ear infection.
- Eli is a monster when he needs to take medicine, spitting everything in mom's face.
- Brett has serious allergies to multiple antibiotics, making it difficult to find a safe medicine that will work.
- Zoe is a twin, and both she and her sister get ear infections when either one of them gets a cold.

- Emerson has had many ear infections already, and it's only October—we expect more ear infections to continue through the winter.
- Aidan is having difficulties with his speech.

Other children have factors that weigh against early placement of tubes:

- Alexa's ear infections make her only mildly grumpy, and respond quickly to amoxicillin every time.
- Eric has had ear infections for the past several months, but it's now April. I'd want to wait and see if fewer ear infections will occur in the warmer months when fewer cold viruses circulate.

Though tubes can help put an end to a recurrent pattern of painful or continuous ear infections, they are often suggested inappropriately for persistent, noninfected fluid in the middle ear. This condition, called "serous otitis media," can follow an acute ear infection or can arise on its own. (It's an unfortunate name. The word looks like "serious," which doesn't describe this condition. Serous just means watery.) Recent research has shown that serous otitis media can safely be watched rather than "cured" with surgical tubes. There are some special cases where tubes

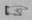 **Ear tubes should not be placed in children who have persistent fluid in their middle ears unless the fluid is causing problems.**

should be considered: a child with speech problems, developmental delay, or other health factors that relate to ear functioning. But in general, children who have fluid behind their eardrums without other symptoms should be managed with observation alone. Your pediatrician should reexamine the ears at routine visits and at any time symptoms seem to be developing.

Follow-up for ear infections is another area of controversy. After a correctly treated and "cured" ear infection, there will often be some residual fluid behind the eardrum. As we've seen, this fluid doesn't hurt anyone, and there is really no reason for the pediatrician to look for it in ordinary children. Unfortunately, the "ear recheck" visit is a routine ritual in many offices, and a big moneymaker too. But once your child is old enough to clearly tell

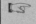 **Ear rechecks are only routinely needed for children under about two years old.**

you when his ears are hurting, there is no reason to return to the office if your child seems fine after completing therapy for an ear infection.

With your insider's knowledge, spot the mistakes that were made in the management of this child:

Molly is three years old and doing well in school. She went to visit her doctor after she twisted her ankle, and at that time yellow fluid was noted behind her eardrum. "Gorillacillin" was prescribed. At her ear recheck visit, a second course of a different antibiotic was given because her eardrum was not normal. After her next abnormal exam a few months later, she was referred to an ENT for placement of ear tubes.

What was wrong with the way Molly was handled?

1. She had no symptoms of an ear infection in the first place, and her eardrum was not red. That means she didn't have an ear infection, and antibiotics should not have been used.
2. Even if she did have an ear infection, because of her age it would have been a good idea to wait before beginning antibiotics.
3. If an antibiotic was needed, amoxicillin should have been used rather than the newer and more expensive "Gorillacillin."
4. Even if she had an ear infection, a three-year-old who has no symptoms doesn't need her ear rechecked.
5. Since she still didn't have symptoms, the subsequent courses of antibiotics were not justified either.
6. Even if she has persistent fluid in the middle ear, a three-year-old doesn't need ear tubes unless the fluid is causing problems.
7. Did anyone do anything about her twisted ankle? That's why she went to the doctor in the first place!

EAR PAIN: WHEN TO CALL

> **!** These red flags mean call your doctor now:
>
> • Your child seems especially ill, uncomfortable, or scared.

Contact your pediatrician during regular hours for a routine appointment to determine the cause and best therapy for a child's ear pain.

The diagnosis and treatment of the common ear infection is not as straightforward as you might guess. Though most doctors mean well, many are not following the best ways of treating and following up on ear infections. Now that you know the inside story, you'll be better able to know when your child does and does not need antibiotics for an ear infection, and how to avoid unnecessary worry, time, and expense.

6

PINK EYE

People notice pink eyes. Day care centers hate them, and shoo children with
even the mildest pink eyes away. Parents want a quick cure to prevent an infectious pink eye spreading throughout the house. Kids who have a red eye from
a scratch can be in tremendous pain, and might not even be able to open their
eyes for an exam. Fortunately, the list of causes of pink eyes is not long, and
parents can quickly learn how to manage most pink eyes without much fuss.
Infection is by far the most common cause of pink eyes in babies and preschoolers. Trauma, allergies, and rare-but-serious other things can also occur.

THE COMMON PINK EYE: CONJUNCTIVITIS

Conjunctivitis means inflammation (in this case, redness) of the outer lining
of the eye. The first tip about di-
agnosing pink eye is simple, but
many day care centers seem to
get this one wrong. I evaluate

> ☞ **Pink eyes are pink.**

many children sent home from day care for "pink eye" whose eyes are perfectly white, but might have some goo in them. These children do not have
pink eye, and if otherwise feeling well should remain in school.

> Three-year-old Alex has been sent home for the third time this April
> with pink eyes. Both of his eyes are watery and light pink, and he is
> rubbing them. He says they're itchy. Though they've recurred despite
> antibiotic drops, no one else in his family has seemed to catch these
> recurrent pink eyes from him.

There are three varieties of conjunctivitis:

Bacterial. Eyes with bacterial infections are more red than pink, and usually filled
with goo. The child usually feels well otherwise, although about one in three

infants with bacterial pink eye will also have an ear infection caused by the same bacteria. These kids are contagious, though they quickly improve with antibiotic eyedrops. They can return to school after twenty-four hours on drops.

Viral. Infectious pink eye in children is about half bacterial, and half viral. The kids with viral conjunctivitis tend to feel a little sicker overall, with perhaps some cold symptoms and fever. Their eyes are more pink than red, and more watery than gooey. Although they're usually put on eyedrops, as with other viral infections antibiotics do not help. Despite drops, kids remain infectious until their overall illness, including fevers, is improved. There is no simple rule for how many days this might take. The only ways to prevent the spread of viral conjunctivitis are to wash hands, avoid sharing towels and linens, and keep children with pink eye isolated.

> ☞ **Though your child may be taking eyedrops, if viral conjunctivitis is the cause he will remain contagious until the eye is no longer pink. The drops don't help.**

Allergic. Allergic conjunctivitis begins simultaneously in both eyes, is more itchy than stingy, and more watery than gooey. Usually kids with allergic conjunctivitis have other allergic symptoms, like sneezing or a congested nose.

So what does Alex have? They're recurrent, simultaneous, and itchy; and they're watery rather than gooey. It's doubtful they're infectious, as no one seems to catch it from him. Alex has allergic conjunctivitis, and he should stay in school.

TREATMENT OF INFECTIONS CONJUNCTIVITIS

If your doctor suspects an infectious conjunctivitis, whether viral or bacterial, antibiotic eyedrops are usually prescribed. Although we know they won't help for the approximately 50 percent of pink eyes that are caused by viruses, it is difficult to know if an infection is definitely viral. Ask your doctor if the pink eye is likely viral or bacterial so you can make plans for day care and potential family transmission.

There are about a dozen different antibiotic eyedrops on the market. The oldest ones tend to be the cheapest, but can be stingy or burny (Sulamyd or Garamycin). More expensive newer agents are more comfortable, including Vigamox, Zymar, and Ocuflox. Brands that are comfortable and available as inexpensive generics include Polytrim and Ciloxan.

> ☞ **Don't even try to open your child's eyes for drops. Just let her lie down, face up; if she screws her eyes shut, that's fine. Put a few drops in a corner of each affected eye, making a little lake. Then blow in your child's face. The eyes pop open, and the drops fall in!**

There isn't an exact dose for antibiotic eyedrops. Use as much as you need to make sure at least one drop falls in. Many ophthalmologists recommend using extra frequent doses on the first day—as frequently as every two hours—to hasten the healing of bacterial conjunctivitis.

Trauma-Related Pink Eye

When the surface of the eye gets scratched it hurts and turns red. Sometimes the history of the trauma is clear—a Dad may know that he accidentally scratched the child's eye with his finger, or the child may complain of eye pain right after a poke with a twig. Other times, the cause of the scratch is known only indirectly. For instance, a child who complains of a pink and painful eye after playing in a sandbox probably has sand in his eye. Other clues that should make a parent suspicious of a scratched rather than infected eye are:

- A single eye that suddenly becomes painful and red.
- A child complains of a feeling like "something is stuck in my eye."
- A child says it hurts when he looks back and forth with his eyes closed.

If your child has had significant trauma, cover the eye with something to keep it dark and protected and seek immediate medical attention. If it is during the day, you can call an ophthalmologist for an exam in the office, or just proceed to the emergency room. Examples of significant trauma would be an eye struck by a batted ball, or an eye injured by glass shards during an automobile accident.

Following a more mild incident, try to flush your child's eye out with tap water, or better yet contact lens saline solution. (You can use saline, or any soaking liquid that is meant to stay on the lens as it is inserted into the eye. Never put contact lens cleaning solution in anyone's eye.) If your child remains in pain or won't tolerate your rinsing out the foreign material, seek medical attention. Scratches across the cornea in the front of the eye can be very painful, and your child may need to be evaluated for strong pain relievers to use while the eye heals. Most minor eye scratches and abrasions can be managed by your pediatrician.

The "Other" Pink Eye

Most pink eyes are caused by infection, allergies, or trauma. But if your child has pink eyes that don't respond to therapy, or include symptoms like distorted vision or severe headaches, you may have an unusual pink eye that needs to be evaluated by an ophthalmologist. If you're not confident that your child's eye has been correctly diagnosed and treated, ask for a specialist's evaluation.

The reddest, most dramatic eye that a parent is likely to see is caused by a "subconjunctival hemorrhage" when there is bleeding underneath the lining of the eye. This can occur after any incident with head squeezing or pressure, most commonly in a newborn after childbirth or in an older child after forceful vomiting. Fortunately, though they look bad these eyes heal well and require no treatment after your pediatrician's evaluation confirms that the bleeding is only under the eye's lining.

PINK EYE: WHEN TO CALL

> ! These red flags mean call your doctor now:
> - Pink eye following significant trauma.
> - Your child seems especially ill, uncomfortable, or scared.

Contact your pediatrician during regular hours for a routine appointment to evaluate and treat ordinary pink eye.

Almost all conjunctivitis is more of a nuisance than a serious infection. Though the day care centers panic at the sight of a pink eye, the common cold causes far more misery—yet kids who are coughing and congested are seldom rushed home. Only a small percentage of pink eyes require ophthalmologic care, but if your child remains symptomatic after ordinary treatment, or has a red eye with changes in vision, seek an ophthalmologist's opinion right away.

7

THE COMMON COLD AND THE FLU

Colds are common. Preschoolers struggle through eight or so a year, even more if they're in group care. As the name suggests, colds occur more often when it's cold. Many kids stay congested all winter, when one cold follows immediately after another. Common they might be, but colds are not easy to treat. There is very little evidence that any medication is likely to relieve the symptoms of cough and congestion in a child. That hasn't stopped a multitude of drug manufacturers from marketing dozens of products to sniffly, feverish children and adults.

A common cold, or "upper respiratory infection," is caused by one of hundreds of different viruses that invade the cells lining the upper respiratory tract: the nose, sinuses, and throat. They spread via droplets of mucus transmitted from an infected person, usually via hands. Colds are more common in winter because people congregate indoors and stay closer to one another.

> ☞ **The most effective way to prevent the transmission of colds is frequent hand washing or use of an alcohol-based hand sanitizer.**

There may be some truth to grandma's advice to bundle up—in the winter, cold air prevents the nose from effectively filtering out viruses. Still, colds are not caused by wet hair or playing outside when it rains. They're caused by viruses spread by other people.

SYMPTOMS

The common cold includes a group of symptoms that follows the same predictable progression in both children and adults:

Day 0–1: A vague feeling of illness, called the prodrome, heralds the onset of a new cold. In babies this is subtle. Older kids and adults might complain of a sense of illness, tingly skin, headache, or a mild scratchy throat. During this phase, the patient is already contagious, but probably doesn't know it yet! Babies and preschoolers are more likely than adults to run a fever during the first few days of a cold.

Day 2–4: Now the throat becomes sore, and any fever should begin to improve.

Day 4–7: The throat is better, but the nose is worse! In this phase, the most bothersome symptom is a stuffy or runny nose. When a child has a brief sore throat preceding a few days of stuffy nose, the diagnosis of a viral cold is clear.

Day 7–14: Cough, cough, cough. This part of the cold can linger for days or weeks, and can really be disruptive for the whole household. By day ten of the cold there is usually significant improvement in the nasal symptoms, but the cough can persist far longer.

TREATMENT

What interventions help for a cold? First, the nonmedicines. These are the safest and most effective ways to help your child feel better:

- Rest helps everyone.
- Offer extra fluids, especially if fever is present. This prevents dehydration and keeps mucus from getting sticky and cloggy.
- Saline nose spray is useful especially in little babies to keep a nose runny and loose rather than all plugged up.
- Steam can also help keep things loose, but don't hold a baby near any source of hot steam. It is safest to sit together in a steamy bathroom.
- Humidifiers also keep the air passages moist. The cool mist ones are safer when Junior accidentally pulls it down onto his head!
- Chicken soup, popsicles, and comfort food are as helpful and important as any medicine during a cold.

What about medicines or herbs that are commonly prescribed or recommended? I've grouped commonly used medicines by type, but keep in mind that many cold medicines are optimistically marketed as combinations of ingredients in "multisymptom cold relievers." A few of the common brands of over-the-counter medicines are listed as examples. There are countless combinations of these. Similar ingredients are sold in prescription versions, too.

Antihistamines (diphenhydramine [Benadryl], brompheniramine, and others found in many combination cold remedies). There is no plausible reason for antihistamines to help with any of the symptoms of the common cold, and no studies have shown antihistamines to help with viral symptoms in children. But they certainly can help some children sleep! That's right: they're used as a sedative, often in combination with other "cold medicines" to counteract the stimulant effect of decongestants. Be careful, as some kids respond to antihistamines by getting hyperactive and agitated. But most children get sleepy if given a medicine containing an antihistamine.

Antipyretics/pain relievers (acetaminophen and ibuprofen, found in Tylenol, Motrin, and Advil). These medicines relieve fevers or the achiness that accompanies many viral infections, and they're the most useful medicines for a cold. Any child who is fussy with a cold should be given some pain-relieving medicine, at least as a trial. Keep giving them if they seem to help. These medicines are very safe if used as directed, but parents need to watch the doses and intervals, especially in an ill or feverish child who may be dehydrated.

Cough suppressants (dextromethorphan [Delsym, Robitussin Pediatric Cough] and narcotics). Dextromethorphan is a mildly effective cough suppressant, available over the counter in many brand and generic products. The more potent cough suppressants are narcotics like codeine, found in virtually all prescription cough medicines. Narcotic cough medicines decrease coughing somewhat—probably because they put your child to sleep. These medicines are sedating at usual doses, and potentially lethal in an overdose. The best time to use a narcotic cough suppressant is at bedtime in children whose coughs are keeping them awake. Antihistamines such as Benadryl are marketed as cough suppressants as well, and may have some mild effectiveness. They also work because they're sedating.

Decongestant nasal sprays (phenylephrine [Neo-Synepherine, Little Noses Decongestant] or oxymetazoline [Afrin]). Unlike the other agents in this list, decongestant nasal sprays can improve symptoms of nasal stuffiness and drip. They are marketed for children ages two and up, and they may be safe when used in younger children (ask your own pediatrician before using any medication that isn't labeled for your child's age.) These agents can also be physically addictive, requiring more frequent administration to prevent ever-worsening rebound congestion. If your child is truly miserable with nasal symptoms, talk to your pediatrician about the safest way to use these topical agents for short-term symptom relief.

Decongestants-oral (pseudoephedrine or phenylephrine, found in Sudafed and many other medications). These supposedly help "dry up" your nose. Well-done studies have found they are not effective, despite their widespread usage.

Decongestants and Regulations in the United States

The decongestant phenylpropanolamine was taken off the market in 2000 because of fears it caused strokes, especially in young women taking high doses as a weight loss remedy. Pseudoephedrine is an in-gredient in the illicit manufacture of methamphetamines, so sales of products that contain pseudoephedrine became legally restricted in 2006. Almost all OTC oral decongestants have now been reformu-lated using phenylephrine, even though this medication is absorbed poorly and has not been well studied in children.

Decongestants can cause jitteriness and sleeplessness. Very serious adverse reactions, including deaths, have been reported from the use of decongestant medications in young babies, so these should be used with caution under age two—and not at all under age one. Bottom line: you can try them for an older child, but be careful about the dose and beware of potential side effects. Only continue using decongestants (or any other cold medication) if they genuinely seem to help your child feel better.

Expectorants (guaifenesin, found in Robitussin and many other products). This one might be hard to swallow, and not just because guaifenesin tastes terrible. There is zero evidence that expectorant medications do anything to lessen any symptoms of a cold. They certainly are safe, though, so if they've seemed to help feel free to continue using them.

> ☞ **The medicines in cold remedies are not effective. The same or similar ingredients are used in both prescription and OTC cold remedies; none of them have been shown to work well in children.**

Antibiotics. If the diagnosis is the common cold or an upper respiratory infection, there is no antibiotic that will make any difference. None. Taking an antibiotic during a cold will also not prevent any complications. Do not take any antibiotics for a common cold; do not pressure the doctor into prescribing one; and if you have a doctor who seems too quick to give out antibiotic prescriptions, you ought to find a new doctor. Some colds can lead to other infections, including ear infections or sinusitis, which *might* benefit from an antibiotic. Or they might not! See the chapters on these other infections for more details about when an antibiotic can genuinely be helpful.

Echinacea. This herb has become popular as both a common cold preventive and cure. There have been some studies in adults showing that administration of echinacea at the start of a cold may reduce the number of days of symptoms, though other studies refute this. Studies in children have not been encouraging. If you wish to try echinacea, it makes more sense to start taking it at the first sign of a cold rather than take it all of the time.

Zinc. At least one study in adults showed that frequent consumption of zinc lozenges beginning at the start of a cold reduced the length of symptoms, though many of the participants dropped out of the study because the zinc made them ill. In the study that showed the best effect, volunteers took zinc lozenges every two hours.

Unfortunately, few medicines are really effective at helping cold symptoms. Some may help your child sleep better—and that is important—but none eliminate any symptoms. As with all medical interventions, their potential benefit must always be weighed against any potential risk. If your child has cold symptoms that really aren't bothersome, I would not suggest any cold medicine at all. It may be worth a trial of medicine if symptoms like cough are keeping your child awake, or if a stuffy nose is making your child fussy or upset.

To recap: if your child has a cold, wash everyone's hands, so no one else gets it. Keep the child away from school, especially for the first few days. Get rest, give fluids, and rely mostly on nonmedical approaches to symptom relief. If your child is uncomfortable, give pain medicine. Expect the congestion to last from seven to ten days, and the cough to linger a bit after that.

During a cold, go see the pediatrician if:

- Fever persists more than three days.
- Pain or fussiness isn't relieved by over-the-counter pain medicine.
- Your child cannot eat nor drink.
- Congestion lingers and causes misery for more than ten days.

- Cough lingers and causes misery for more than fourteen days.
- For any reason your child seems more ill than you expect for a cold.

INFLUENZA

Influenza, or "the flu," is a term used informally to mean different things. A brief illness with vomiting is often called a "stomach flu," and sometimes bad winter colds are called "the flu." But in fact neither an illness with mostly vomiting nor a "bad cold" are likely to truly be influenza.

The influenza virus infects people of all ages, usually in the winter. Symptoms start with a vaguely unwell feeling, followed by the rapid development of fever and chills. The fever can be quite high—perhaps 105° F. Often, there are body aches and headaches. Respiratory symptoms like sore throat, runny nose, and cough are usually not severe. Sometimes abdominal pain, vomiting, or diarrhea can occur. Rare complications include pneumonia, shock, seizures, problems with the liver or heart, or overwhelming secondary infections. Each year, about 36,000 people die from influenza in the United States, making it the most common vaccine-preventable cause of death in this country. Influenza is very contagious, and will often strike several family members one after another.

Prevention of influenza begins with hygiene and careful hand washing, as reviewed in Chapter 1. People ill with fever should not attend work or day care, especially in the winter during flu epidemics. Influenza vaccines are safe and effective, and should be given yearly to all children age five and under (plus many other children in high-risk groups). The first year your infant gets a flu vaccine, the dose should be repeated after one month to get the best protective effect. Although a small number of people will get a little achy or feverish after a flu vaccine, the vaccine itself cannot in any way transmit the actual flu disease. Ask anyone who really had genuine flu: the disease is far, far worse than the rare side effects of the vaccine.

Influenza treatment includes all of the supportive measures listed under the common cold. Fevers can be controlled with acetaminophen or ibuprofen; aspirin should be avoided because it can trigger a fatal liver disease called Reye Syndrome if taken during an influenza infection. Although there are some medications that can help a child fight through a flu infection, these do not work dramatically well and need to be started early in the infection to be effective. Children who develop flu are not immune from future infections, and should continue to be vaccinated in future years.

COLDS AND FLU: WHEN TO CALL

> **!** These red flags mean call your doctor now:
> - Your child is having difficulty breathing.
> - Your child seems especially ill, uncomfortable, or scared.

Flu makes children and their parents truly miserable, and can lead to severe complications and death. It is difficult to treat, but can be prevented. Both influenza and the common cold are caused by viruses that can cause a great deal of misery for your children. Because medicines to treat these viral infections are largely ineffective, prevention is the best strategy.

8

SINUSITIS

One of the most common reasons for a sick visit to a pediatrician is nasal congestion and stuffiness. Though this is usually caused by cold viruses or allergies, occasionally mucus that persists in the upper nose can become infected by bacteria. This infection, which always comes after a period of ordinary congestion, is commonly called sinusitis or a "sinus infection." Though technically sinusitis can be caused by allergy, bacteria, viruses, or other infections, most doctors use this term only for *bacterial* infections of the sinuses. In truth, nearly identical symptoms can be triggered by the other causes, and telling the difference between the causes of sinus symptoms is not straightforward. Every parent of a congested child should try to make sure that the best therapy is available to help their child feel better.

Sinus cavities are not opened up at birth, but develop over childhood. It is very uncommon to see genuine sinus infections in the very young. However, they can certainly occur in preschool-aged children.

How Sinus Infections Develop

Ordinarily, the sinus cavities themselves are sterile—no germs are supposed to live in there. Nearby in the nose, though, all sorts of bacteria and viruses may be present. These are ordinarily kept out of the sinuses by several overlapping and very effective mechanisms:

- Sticky mucus is secreted by the cells lining the sinuses, which makes it difficult for germs to attach. However, in some children this mucus can't be cleared out easily. Any stagnant pool of warm mucus will eventually turn into a breeding ground for bacteria. This occurs in children who anatomically have poor drainage of their sinuses (this runs in families), or in children with conditions like cystic fibrosis.

- Immune cells, with the help of antibodies secreted into mucus, attack and fight off any germ invaders. But people with poor immune systems may not be able to rely on this.
- Little hairs called "cilia" push mucus up and out of the sinus cavities. This acts like a constant conveyor belt to move out germs and debris. Kids who live with smokers have impaired cilia, and get more sinus infections.

Sinus infections always begin with some condition leading to excessive sticky mucus, like a viral cold or allergy. Once the nose is stuffed up, the sinuses can't drain properly. And the warm mucus sitting there day after day becomes an inviting target for bacterial invaders.

> ☞ **Sinus infections begin *after* the nose has been congested for at least several days.**

PREVENTION

The most effective way to prevent sinus infections is to prevent the viral infections that trigger them. Washing hands frequently and avoiding sick people are the best strategies (see Chapter 1). Also, avoid and treat allergies that cause chronic nasal congestion.

When your child does have a cold, use simple and effective measures to help clear the mucus. Keep children well hydrated with plenty of fluids, and keep the air humid. This prevents mucus from getting thick and sticky. Warm steam can help mobilize the mucus, but be careful with younger children to avoid burns. Nasal saline drops or spray can be used at any age to help clear out the nose.

You might expect that cold medicines—that is, medicines that are marketed to reduce congestion—would prevent a cold from turning into a sinus infection. However, this isn't the case. Using decongestants, antihistamines, expectorants, or any combination of these does *not* reduce your child's chance of developing a sinus infection from a cold. For more details about cold medicines and their use, see Chapter 7.

> ☞ **You can't rely on medicines to prevent sinus infections.**

DIAGNOSIS

Eleven-month-old Kira developed cold symptoms about two weeks ago. At first, she had a fever and a poor appetite. She then developed a runny nose, followed by a cough. Though it's been two weeks, her cough isn't improving—in fact, it seems to be getting worse! And that nose? It's still thick and running. Kira has been a good sport through most of this, but for the past few days she's been especially fussy and has had trouble sleeping.

What we really want to know: Does Kira have a bacterial infection that will benefit from antibiotics? This is an important question—antibiotic overuse has led to a disastrous rise in bacterial "superbugs" that resist ordinary antibiotics. Antibiotics themselves can also cause significant side effects including severe or deadly allergic reactions. You and your doctor should take the time to be sure of what you're treating before reaching for an antibiotic.

In medicine, the "gold standard" is the absolute best way to diagnose something. To *really* know what's causing sinus congestion, a doctor would need to put a needle into a sinus cavity to collect the mucus for study. Though this is rarely done in ordinary practice, these procedures have been done in research volunteers. Years of experience from pediatricians, infectious disease specialists, and sinus surgeons have also contributed to our understanding of sinusitis. We know what features in the child's illness are likely to mean bacteria, and what features are likely to mean virus. We also know that some features don't really mean either one.

Color of the mucus: Study after study has confirmed that the color of the nasal mucus alone doesn't correlate with either bacterial or viral infections. I know the "common wisdom" is that green or yellow mucus means bacterial infection—but this common wisdom is wrong, and it's been proven to be wrong for years. Mucus that's perfectly clear can occur in a child with a bacterial sinusitis, and mucus that's green and thick can occur in a child with a viral infection. The color itself really doesn't help distinguish the two.

A Science Experiment

Next time you have an ordinary cold with lots of clear mucus, blow your nose into a tissue and save it. The next day, you'll see that the clear mucus has turned into all sorts of lovely colors. Mucus will become thick and dark and green, whether there is a bacterial infection or not. That's why you'll often notice your child's early-morning runny nose is so thick and green—it's been sitting up his nose all night!

Fever: Many viral infections start with a fever, and fevers during the first few days of a congestion illness do not mean any bacteria are present. However, if your child has a cold with a fever that goes away and later comes back, he may well have crossed into a bacterial infection. Fevers are not expected toward the end of an ordinary viral illness.

Other symptoms: Cough, sneezing, and other symptoms of the common cold do not help distinguish between a viral and bacterial sinus infection.

Headache or facial pain: Though these symptoms, especially if severe, do correlate with bacterial sinus infections in older children and adults, they seldom occur in preschoolers.

Misery: Studies in adults have been inconsistent, in part because it is difficult to judge how severe symptoms are. However, it seems true that more severe symptoms, especially if persistent throughout the day, can correlate somewhat with an increased likelihood of bacterial sinusitis.

Timing. I've saved the best for last: the timing of the symptoms is the single best discriminatory factor. An ordinary cold should include congestion that lasts from seven to ten days. Congestion that lasts longer than this, especially if it is worsening after fourteen days, is likely to be caused by a bacterial infection. This makes sense: we know that sinus infections need time to develop, and always occur *after* a child has already been congested for some other reason.

The best way for you and your pediatrician to decide if your congested child needs antibiotics is to look at how long the symptoms have been present, and whether the child is comfortable. For otherwise healthy children, I usually suggest antibiotics for a child whose congestion is uncomfortable and not improving *after* seven to ten days. In a child who feels well, it is reasonable to wait longer to see if the infection will get better on its own.

Can the diagnosis of a sinus infection be confirmed by a radiologist? Unfortunately, the tests for sinus infections are not as useful as you'd think. Plain x-rays are very unreliable in preschoolers, who have small sinus cavities that are difficult to see. CT scans can be used, but these "overcall" sinusitis—that is, they often show mucus that is incorrectly called sinusitis when, in fact, it is merely part of a viral cold. CT scans are most useful for children that have recurring or difficult to treat sinus problems. Both CT scans and x-rays will expose your child to some radiation, and CT scanning usually requires sedation in preschoolers.

TREATMENT

Treatment begins with addressing the symptoms that are bothering the child. Nasal congestion should be first treated with saline drops, extra fluids, and humidity; popsicles and lollipops can help soothe a cough or sore throat. Treat fever or pain with acetaminophen or ibuprofen.

"Cold remedy" medicines will not prevent an ordinary cold from turning into a sinus infection. In fact, they may not be very effective at ameliorating the symptoms of congestion either. There may be significant side effects of cold medications, especially those that contain decongestants. These products may be dangerous if used under age two. But if your older child seems to feel better after administration of a cold medicine (a decongestant, antihistamine, or a combination of the two), then continue to use these. Cough suppressants may also help, especially if the child is having trouble sleeping. See Chapter 7 for further details about the risks, benefits, and safest ways to use cold medicines.

If you and your pediatrician agree that the congestion is caused by a bacterial infection, think about whether an antibiotic is necessary. Most bacterial sinus infections will clear on their own without antibiotics, and in fact the best most recent studies of sinusitis in children have shown that in most circumstances antibiotics help only a little, if at all. If you do decide to proceed with antibiotics, it is best to go with an older, safer, less expensive medicine like amoxicillin. No study has ever shown any other antibiotic to be more effective in treating sinusitis. When taking antibiotics, complete the entire course and take every dose on time as best as possible. More information about common antibiotics used in pediatrics is in Chapter 2.

Some children with sinus problems benefit from a more thorough evaluation, often performed with the help of an ear, nose, and throat specialist. Ask your pediatrician about a specialty referral if your child has significant other health problems, recurring sinus infections (more than three per year), sinus infections that are difficult to clear, or sinus infections that have led to complications.

9

COUGH AND CROUP

Coughs are aggravating. Though a cough itself is a helpful reflex to clear mucus out of the respiratory tract, a child with a bad cough will annoy his classmates and keep a whole family awake. Unfortunately, medicine doesn't work very well at suppressing a child's cough. An occasional sleepless night with your child is the price parents pay for exposures to the hundreds of viruses that trigger most coughs.

CAUSES

Any irritation of the airway, from deep in the lungs to the back of the throat, will make a child cough. In pediatrics, cough is almost always triggered by minor viral infections. These infections can linger a long time. When common cold viruses are given to volunteers under experimental conditions, the cough part of their illness can last for over three weeks!

Bronchitis in children is a poorly defined condition, and means different things to different doctors and patients. As far as I can tell (and this is a *big* secret) it seems to mean "a cough illness for which the doctor or patient wants antibiotics." As is clearly established by multiple studies and every important clinical guideline, a cough illness characterized as "bronchitis" should not be treated with antibiotics. These infections are viral, and antibiotics are much more likely to do harm than good.

There is a different disease in elderly smokers called "chronic bronchitis." This is in part caused by an overgrowth of lung bacteria, and often requires antibiotics. Because our patients have healthy lung tissues, there is no similar condition in pediatrics.

Though it has a similar name, "bronchiolitis" is different from bronchitis. Bronchiolitis is a disease unique to young children, and isn't seen past age two. In bronchiolitis, a cough is accompanied by a tight, wheezy chest. It is triggered by a number of different viral infections, most commonly Respiratory Syncytial Virus (RSV). Bronchiolitis affects the youngest babies most, especially babies who are premature or otherwise ill. Though many medicines have been tried, the best-researched clinical guidelines suggest that the only effective treatment is good supportive care: hydration, nutrition, and looking out for any signs of deterioration or more serious difficulty breathing.

Pneumonia, an infection of the lungs, is an uncommon cause of cough. There are different types. A "lobar pneumonia," named after how it looks on a chest x-ray, is the most serious. Kids with this pneumonia have fevers and are ill, and often complain of chest pain. A "walking pneumonia" is a milder bacterial infection that is rarely seen below age five. The most common kind of pneumonia seen in younger children is caused by viral infections that don't improve with antibiotics. It can be difficult to know for sure if a child with pneumonia has a viral or bacterial infection, so antibiotics are usually prescribed for any sort of pneumonia in children.

Another bacterial infection that can include cough as a symptom is sinusitis. In addition to the cough, symptoms include persistent nasal discharge or stuffiness lasting longer than ten days. Sinusitis rarely presents with cough alone.

Children suffering from allergies will sometimes have cough along with other allergic symptoms: nasal drip or congestion, sneezing, and eye irritation.

A very important diagnosis in childhood that includes cough as a prominent symptom is asthma (see Chapter 10). Though often presenting with cough alone, asthma can also cause shortness of breath, wheezy breathing noises, chest pain, or abdominal pain.

Croup is a cough illness caused by a viral infection of the upper airway, right around the vocal cords. Kids with croup have a unique cough that sounds like a barking seal. Many families refer to all sorts of deep or "bad" coughs as "croupy," but to a doctor this word is reserved for the unique barky seal cough of croup. More about croup appears at the end of this chapter.

Smoking is a common cause of cough. Even when parents only smoke outside, enough smoke can cling to clothes to trigger or prolong a cough in some children.

Some rarer causes of cough include: acid reflux, congenital problems of the lungs or upper airway, drug reactions, inhaled foreign objects, and household exposures to chemicals. Unusual conditions should be more aggressively pursued if an unexplained cough lasts longer than three to six weeks.

Many coughs are self-perpetuating. That is, the child coughs... which irritates the throat, causing more cough ... which further irritates the throat! This vicious cycle can be frustrating and difficult to interrupt, and can make treatment of coughing difficult.

How to Treat a Cough: What Works and What Doesn't

First, try to treat any underlying condition. A child who has asthma leading to cough should have the asthma treated, not the cough suppressed. That being said, most coughs do not have an underlying treatable cause . . . so what can you do for the garden variety, viral-associated cough?

Nonmedical interventions like a humidifier, soothing lollipops, or a popsicle can help. If your child has a barky, croup-like cough in the winter, going outside to breathe cold air can quickly improve croup symptoms. For any sort of cough, warm steam from a shower can be effective. Some people swear by mentholated rubs and vapors; though good studies of these are lacking, if used correctly they're harmless and may be worth a try. (Young children should never be allowed to play with or swallow vapor rubs.) Some children get upset and panic with a bad cough. For them, distraction with a favorite video can be the best "medicine."

There are a few prescription and nonprescription medicines that might help with cough. These are reviewed in Chapter 7.

Most coughs are not caused by serious illnesses. Seek medical attention quickly for any cough accompanied by high fever or shortness of breath. For an ordinary cough illness, home treatment for at least a week or so is the best option. Coughs rarely benefit from antibiotic therapy, but many other medical and nonmedical interventions can help relieve this annoying symptom.

Chronic Cough

Some coughs linger. Though an ordinary viral cough can certainly stick around for three weeks, a cough that's lasting much longer may need more evaluation. What's the next step, and who needs a big specialist work up?

> Four-year-old Cristina has had a cough for six weeks. It seemed to start with an ordinary cold, but the nasal congestion and fever are long gone. She's missed a few days of school, but otherwise seems to feel well—she's full of energy and bouncing around the exam room! Cristina's mom, who works in a hospital, was recently treated with medication when she tested positive for tuberculosis exposure.

Before getting too worried, ask yourself if the cough is serious, or not-so-serious. These questions can help decide if an in-depth evaluation needs to be aggressively pursued:

- Does the cough interfere with normal activity? (For instance, can the child no longer play soccer?)
- Does the cough interfere with the child's sleep?

- Are there unusual exposures to animals, foreign travel, sick people, occupational chemicals, or anything else?
- Are there signs of a more serious illness—fever for more than five days, weight loss, or night sweats?

If some of these red flags are present, get in touch with your doctor for an evaluation to look for the most serious things first. Fortunately, most children with a chronic cough fit into the "not-so-serious," but "nonetheless-getting-to-be-a-nuisance" category. For these children, reviewing a detailed history of the illness and a physical exam with your pediatrician is much more likely to yield an answer than any tests. After this evaluation, try therapy for the most likely diagnosis; if that doesn't work, try the next most likely approach. Though moving step-by-step in this fashion can be frustrating for some families, invasive tests for children who have a benign but chronic cough are unlikely to get you to the finish line any faster.

In our story, Cristina's physician tested her for tuberculosis. This test was negative, and over the next week or so her cough gradually disappeared. Because she was otherwise well, her parents felt comfortable waiting it out a little longer before doing any more invasive tests.

CROUP: WHAT IS IT?

Croup is a viral infection that causes swelling of the upper airway, near the vocal cords. In an adult, this area is wider, so swelling only causes a hoarse voice called "laryngitis." But in a young child, especially less than two, swelling up near the vocal cords causes a unique, seal-like barky cough. If it's more severe, the child will make a high-pitched, squeaky sound when she inhales. The cough and respiratory difficulty of croup is almost always worse at night.

Classic croup is triggered by one of several different respiratory viruses, most usually parainfluenza. (Parainfluenza virus doesn't have much to do with influenza virus. It's just a similar name.) It occurs most commonly in the winter. As with other respiratory viral infections, symptoms like runny nose, nasal congestion, and fever accompany the croup cough. In fact, if a child has a sudden onset of a croup cough without any other symptoms of a viral infection, be a little suspicious that something else is going on—perhaps he is choking on a toy or is having an allergic reaction.

Some children seem to have recurrent bouts of croup. This is sometimes seen in children who are born with a small or floppy upper airway. Another common underlying cause of a recurring croup-like illness is asthma. Your pediatrician, by taking a careful history, should be able to figure this out. Sometimes, referral to an ENT (ear, nose, and throat) or a pulmonary specialist will be necessary.

Prevention of croup requires prevention of the spread of respiratory viruses, primarily through careful and frequent hand washing. See Chapter 1 for more about preventing the viral infections that cause croup and most other coughs from spreading in homes and school.

Croup is usually diagnosed clinically. If a child has upper respiratory symptoms plus the unique croup cough with an otherwise unremarkable exam, it's unnecessary to confirm the diagnosis with any further tests. If the diagnosis is unclear, or the child is especially ill, sometimes an x-ray of the neck or chest can be helpful. It is also possible to test for some of the respiratory viruses that trigger croup by collecting nasal mucus. If croup occurs during an influenza epidemic, this can be especially useful. Unlike the other respiratory viruses, there are specific medicines that can be given to help fight off an influenza infection.

CROUP: TREATMENT

The goal of treatment is to ease the swelling of the upper airway. Try simple measures first: a soothing popsicle, or a lollipop for older kids. Breathing in cold air really helps—if it's winter, go outside or lean with your child out of a window on the ground floor. If it's not cold outside, you can even try breathing the air from a freezer. Warm steam also seems to help, so try sitting in the bathroom with the shower running. Do *not* hold your baby near boiling water or a tea kettle.

There can be a psychological component to croup. Many people get tightness in the throat when they're upset or anxious, and some children will develop this when they're scared and upset with croup. Keep your cool and don't get your child any more excited. Pop in a favorite video to help everyone relax.

> ☞ **Fear and excitement make croup worse. Try to keep your child calm.**

If your child has asthma, try a treatment with rescue medication (usually inhaled albuterol or Xopenex [levalbuterol]). It can be hard to tell if a child is wheezing during a croup-like episode, and a single breathing treatment won't hurt.

Over-the-counter cold medicines have very little effect on croup, but you can try a dose of cough suppressant like dextromethorphan (Delsym, Robitussin Pediatric Cough, or others).

If your child seems to be having difficulty breathing, or is making a squeaky noise, contact your pediatrician. You may need to head to the nearest emergency room for a breathing treatment with epinephrine. Oral or injected steroid medicines can be very effective in opening the swollen airway, but they do not work quickly in an emergency. If you've seen your pediatrician and she's prescribed oral steroids, start taking them right away—do not wait to see if your child has another rough night.

Cough and Croup: When to Call

> ! Contact your pediatrician right away if:
>
> - Your child is having difficulty breathing.
> - Your child looks blue.
> - Your child seems especially ill, uncomfortable, or scared.

Contact your pediatrician during regular hours if:

- A mild cough or croup isn't improving after ten days.
- Your child has recurrent coughing associated with exercise or another particular exposure.
- Your child has had recurrent bouts of croup.

Though coughing is part of many viral illnesses, it will usually go away on its own. Beware of kids who are having trouble breathing during their cough, and look out for the few kids whose cough don't fit the typical reassuring viral pattern. Patience and simple home remedies are the best ways to help most children get over a cough.

10

WHEEZING AND ASTHMA

Rachel's parents are worried. Their three-month-old baby girl had been well until five days ago, when she developed an ordinary cold with nasal congestion and an occasional cough. Today, they've noticed her breathing is labored and noisy. Her chest seems to cave in with every breath, and her grandmother thinks she is wheezing.

Common colds are common. But some babies take ordinary viral respiratory infections a step further—they develop trouble breathing, with wheezy respirations and labored chest wall movements. They have to use the muscles between their ribs to get a good breath, and you can see the effort. Once the cold virus passes, breathing returns to normal. Unfortunately, many babies who wheeze once during a cold are likely to wheeze repeatedly during every common cold.

For parents, this can be a frustrating dilemma. They know that colds trigger wheezing, but colds are very hard to avoid in preschoolers, especially among children in group care. Furthermore, medicines for wheezing may not be very effective in babies. Reading and learning about wheezing in infants can be difficult, as different doctors use different words to discuss this problem.

DEFINITIONS

Wheezing and asthma are confusing topics—even to many doctors. We need to first agree on what we're talking about.

Common cold. Triggered by one of many different respiratory viruses, the common cold causes sore throat, nasal congestion, and a mild cough that can persist for a few weeks. Common colds are more common in the winter, and are very contagious. For more information, see Chapter 7.

Wheezing. This is an abnormal noise made while exhaling through narrowed tubes in the lungs. You can probably imitate a wheeze noise by tightening your throat and exhaling. Sometimes, babies who are wheezing will have noisy inhalations, too. Although wheezing is best heard through a stethoscope, if it is severe you can hear it across a room. Lung tubes can be narrowed when they are lined with mucus, or when the muscle walls around them constrict.

Bronchiolitis. Only seen in infants, bronchiolitis is a viral infection of the airways in the lungs. It causes wheezing plus ordinary cold symptoms. In the winter, it is usually triggered by respiratory syncytial virus (RSV). Bronchiolitis can occur more than once in the same child, but if it is recurrent the child is usually thought of as having asthma.

Bronchitis. Though the name looks similar, bronchitis is not the same as bronchiolitis. Bronchitis specifically refers to a chronic inflammatory and infectious disorder in elderly smokers, though it is sometimes used as a looser term in otherwise healthy adults with a bad cough. The term should really be avoided as it lacks a good consistent meaning from doctor to doctor. "Recurrent bronchitis" in children is asthma, even if the doctor is reluctant to use that term.

Asthma. Asthma means recurring bouts of reversible airway obstruction, usually manifested as wheezing. In adults and teenagers, the wheezy episodes often have a variety of triggers: exercise, cold air, respiratory infections, environmental pollutants, and others. In preschool and younger kids, the wheezy episodes are almost always triggered by common colds. This and other differences have led many doctors to question whether recurrent wheezing in adults and babies is really the same illness. For now, we seem stuck using the same word: asthma. Some experts suggest pediatricians use a different term, such as "recurrent viral-induced wheezing of childhood." That tongue twister is unlikely to catch on!

CAUSES AND PREVENTION

A wheezing noise is caused by airway narrowing, triggered by either mucus or the constriction of tiny muscles around the airway. Exactly why some children have bouts of wheezing is unclear, but there are probably multiple contributing factors.

Certain viruses are much more likely to invade the lungs and trigger wheezing. The main culprit is RSV or respiratory syncytial virus. This usually circulates in the wintertime, and in most children and adults causes a common cold with symptoms similar to any other cold. But in some newborns and babies, RSV triggers inflammation in the lungs which results in wheezing. Babies who have had an RSV infection with wheezing are more likely to continue having recurrent wheezing as children, and more likely to have genuine asthma as adults. What is unclear is whether the RSV is the chicken or the egg. Did the RSV damage or change the lungs permanently, leading to asthma, or are babies who are destined to develop asthma more likely to wheeze when they get an RSV infection?

Genetics and the environment certainly play important roles. Asthma often occurs in multiple family members, and often occurs in individuals who have other so-called "atopic" diseases: allergic rhinitis (hay fever), food allergies, and eczema. It's clear that there is more asthma in developed countries. Environmental pollutants like ozone and smog can trigger asthma flare-ups in susceptible people, but there is little evidence that pollution actually causes asthma.

While asthma and other atopic diseases are becoming more frequent in the developed world, it is less clear what families can do to prevent it. Though there are other good reasons to breastfeed and avoid day care, studies of these strategies have not consistently proven that they prevent asthma. RSV infections seem to predispose children to future asthma, but these are very contagious and difficult to avoid. Strategies to reduce early exposures to common allergy triggers have not consistently been shown to prevent either allergy or asthma. Tobacco exposure is a definite risk factor for asthma, so a reasonable step to prevent the development of asthma in your children is to avoid tobacco smoke both during and after pregnancy.

SYMPTOMS

While wheezing is the defining physical sign of asthma, the most common symptom reported by parents is cough. The cough itself can be wet, dry, or anywhere in between. It tends to be worse at night. Some parents hear a "wheezy" nature to an asthmatic cough.

> ☞ **In babies and children, the most common trigger of an asthmatic episode is a common cold.**

In babies and preschoolers, wheezing episodes almost always occur during or just after an ordinary cold. A typical story that I hear from parents is that their child's colds are always accompanied by a bad cough that takes weeks to clear. Recurring episodes like this make me suspect asthma, even if I don't hear wheezing during a physical exam.

Do Children with Asthma Always Wheeze? Do They Always Cough?

Asthma means periodic, recurrent bouts of airway obstruction, followed by a return to normal lung functioning. Though an obstructed airway will almost always make a wheezy sound as a child exhales, some children are very sensitive to the sensation of tightness in the chest. These kids cough to "force open" the lungs, even before a doctor or parent could have heard the wheezing. This is sometimes called "cough-variant" asthma.

Coughing is a natural reflex. It will occur in anyone whose nervous system can sense mucus in their lungs or any resistance to exhalation.

The cough reflex will help expel mucus, and can at least temporarily "stretch out" air tubes that had been constricted tight.

Both coughing and wheezing are *almost* always present in a child during an episode of asthma.

Diagnosis

The diagnosis of a wheezy episode is based on the history and physical exam. Sometimes, a nasal mucus sample can be tested for respiratory viruses including RSV, though this doesn't change the way the illness is treated.

Asthma is a clinical diagnosis, based on a history of recurring bouts of wheezy illness. Lung function testing is unreliable in babies, though it can be helpful in the diagnosis and ongoing follow-up of asthma in older children. A chest x-ray can exclude other problems, but cannot confirm asthma or wheezing.

Pediatricians often rely on a child's response to asthma medicines to help corroborate the diagnosis of asthma. If your child has a bad or recurrent cough that reliably and consistently improves with the medicines listed later in the chapter, it's asthma.

Treatment

There are two kinds of medicine for asthma or wheezing: the first group are called "rescue medicines," and are used to treat active symptoms. The second group are called "controllers," and are used to *prevent* the next bout of wheezing. If your child is wheezing, coughing, or short of breath, the most important medicines are the rescue medicines. Controller medicines are meant to be used every day, consistently, as a preventive strategy. It's very important that parents treating asthma understand which medicine is to be used during an emergency.

The goals of asthma treatment should be:

1. Preventing and treating symptoms, like cough and shortness of breath.
2. Keeping a child active and able to participate in ordinary play and activities.
3. Preventing severe flare-ups that require oral steroids and trips to the emergency room.

With these in mind, asthma therapy can be tailored to each individual child. Many kids have only mild, occasional flare-ups that coincide with colds. These children can rely on using their rescue medicines alone every once in a while. Other children have more frequent or severe flares, and need to stay on daily medicines. Be sure to follow up with your pediatrician so she can get to know your own child's pattern and the best way for you to use these medicines.

If your child has a history of recurrent wheezing and develops a cough, don't hesitate to start the rescue medications. Treating a flare early can prevent kids from getting sicker, and can keep you out of the emergency room! If you do find that you're having to use the rescue medicines more than once a week (on average), you should meet with your pediatrician to see if a controller medicine should be added.

How to Give Inhaled Medicines to a Child

Ideal medicines for wheezing are inhaled, so they go directly to the lungs. This is the best way to get a high concentration of medication exactly where you need it, getting the most benefit with the fewest side effects. In young children, inhaled medicines are usually given with the help of one of these devices:

- A nebulizer, which is an air compressor attached to a chamber of medication. The compressed air forces the medicine into a mist that the child inhales, usually over five to ten minutes. It's pretty foolproof, though you have to get the child to keep the mask on—waving the mask in front of him will not deliver the medication well.
- A mask-spacer, which is attached to the medicine in a small aerosol can. Teens and adults often use the aerosol can alone, without a spacer; but babies and children have a tough time getting the breathing in sync with the device, and using a spacer makes this easy. A common brand of mask-spacer is called an Aerochamber with Mask. If one of these is prescribed, a doctor or nurse should show you how to use it correctly. It's simple, but easier to show than explain. A single spacer device can be swapped out and used with multiple medications.

MEDICATIONS FOR WHEEZING AND ASTHMA

Albuterol (Ventolin or Proventil; also called Salbutamol). Albuterol is the main rescue medicine for asthma and wheezing. It is available as an inexpensive generic, and can be given through a nebulizer machine or through a mask-spacer device. It is most effective when used occasionally and intermittently. If used even once a day for extended periods of time, albuterol will lose its effectiveness. Anyone who needs to use albuterol frequently needs to try other medications as controllers, saving the albuterol for flare-ups. In fact, frequent and inappropriate use of albuterol is a risk factor for death from asthma—people who've become less responsive to albuterol because of overuse have no good emergency medicine to fall back on when they really get sick. Though albuterol is available as an oral medicine in syrup or pill form, these are much less effective and more prone to side effects. Some, but not most, kids get jittery after inhaled albuterol. This effect usually fades within a few minutes.

Levalbuterol (Xopenex). Albuterol's fancy brand-name cousin is Xopenex. As a rescue medicine, it is just as effective as albuterol. Whether or not it actually works a little better is controversial. Xopenex may have the advantage of somewhat fewer side effects than albuterol. If your child seems especially prone to jitteriness after albuterol, the extra cost of Xopenex may be justified. Like albuterol, Xopenex can be given through a nebulizer machine or mask-spacer.

Fluticasone (Flovent). A steroid controller medicine only available for use with a mask-spacer device, Flovent has minimal side effects and can safely prevent asthma flare-ups. Usually, the lowest dose form (44 mcg per puff) is used in younger children. The only side effect you're likely to see is oral thrush, which can be prevented by having the child sip a few gulps of water after each use. Although FDA-labeled for twice-a-day use, Flovent can be very effective when used just once a day. There are other very similar inhaled steroids available for mask-spacer use, including Qvar and Azmacort.

Budesonide (Pulmicort). Similar in use, effectiveness, and side effects to Flovent, Pulmicort is another inhaled steroid used as a controller medicine. It has to be given through a nebulizer machine once or twice a day.

Montelukast (Singulair). This is a unique, nonsteroid controller medicine that is usually taken as a chewable tablet once a day. A packet of Singulair "sprinkles" is also available, but it's easier to crush the chewables. Head-to-head, Singulair is not as effective in controlling recurrent wheezing as are the inhaled steroids Flovent and Pulmicort.

Prednisone or Prednisolone (Orapred, Prelone). These are oral steroids taken during severe asthma flare-ups. Although they're very effective at stopping asthma symptoms, significant and serious side effects can occur if oral steroids are taken frequently. If your child needs a five-day course of oral steroids more than twice a year to control asthma flare-ups, you should talk to your doctor about using daily controller medicines.

Should You Be Scared of Steroids?

Oral steroids, including prednisone, can be lifesaving in a severe asthma flare-up; they can also be necessary to halt long-standing wheezing or wheezing that doesn't improve with albuterol. But the side effects of frequent use can include problems with growth, blood pressure, cataracts, ulcers, and many other difficulties. One goal of asthma management should be to avoid the use of oral steroids as much as possible.

Inhaled steroids are a different story. These medicines are only barely absorbed into the body, and are rapidly deactivated by the liver before they can cause side effects. If your child has frequent or severe wheezing, don't hesitate to use inhaled steroids—they're the most effective asthma controller medicines available.

ASTHMA AND WHEEZING: WHEN TO CALL

> !   These red flags mean call your doctor now:
>
> - Your child is having difficulty breathing, speaking, or eating.
> - For children who are being treated for wheezing, call if you can still hear wheezing after giving your child rescue medication.
> - Your child looks blue.
> - Your child seems especially ill, uncomfortable, or scared.

Contact your pediatrician during regular hours for a routine appointment if:

- You don't see improvement in wheezing within twenty-four hours of starting your child's rescue medication.
- You've been consistently needing to use rescue medication more than four treatments per month.

Wheezy illnesses are common in babies and children, and if the pattern of wheezing is recurrent it is called asthma. Though we don't understand the best way to prevent asthma from developing, we do have good, safe medication to treat it. Treatment involves both taking care of the immediate problem and sometimes using controller medicines to prevent future wheezing episodes. Work with your pediatrician to develop a prevention and treatment action plan so you can best help your child.

11

ABDOMINAL PAIN

Most bellyaches in preschoolers have no serious cause and will go away on their own. However, every once in a while a more significant problem causes belly pain that needs to be evaluated and treated urgently. Although there are far too many causes of abdominal pain to review extensively in this chapter, every parent should be able to use some insider knowledge to know when belly pain is something to worry about.

SYMPTOMS

Abdominal pain in preschoolers can usually be diagnosed by the history—that is, the story of how the abdominal pain occurs. Keep track of the history carefully, so you can accurately discuss your child's case with the pediatrician. We want to know:

- How long has this been going on? Has it been daily or intermittent?
- When does it hurt? This includes time of day and days of the week, but also how episodes of pain relate to meals, bowel movements, activities, and other things going on in the child's life.
- Where does it hurt? Ask you child to point with one finger. Ask, "Does it hurt anywhere else?"
- Do meals, medicines, or anything else make it better or worse?
- Are there other symptoms that accompany the pain, like vomiting, diarrhea, or heartburn? How about fevers, headaches, painful urination, or anything else?

Pain lasting more than two weeks is called "chronic." The historical information listed above becomes even more crucial to reaching an accurate diagnosis. If your child is having persistent abdominal pain you should keep track of the details in a journal to share with your pediatrician.

Talking about the pain and exploring the cause can itself be therapeutic. For more information about how to talk about symptoms with your child, see Chapter 23.

Often, parents feel that their newborns are having belly pain or cramps. When little babies get upset, they draw their legs up and tense their bellies—but this doesn't mean their bellies hurt, or even that they're having pain at all. It's just that they have a very limited number of ways to express themselves. Though sometimes food intolerance, constipation, or other things can cause abdominal pain in little babies, don't be too quick to assume that fussing newborns have anything wrong in their bellies. For guidance about evaluating a newborn who seems to be having bellyaches, see Chapter 19.

ACUTE ABDOMINAL PAIN: CAUSES

Pain lasting less than two weeks is usually triggered by a mild infection. Sometimes there are no other symptoms, but often a mild fever, congestion, cough, headache, vomiting, or diarrhea will accompany the pain. If these symptoms are not too disturbing to your child, you're probably dealing with a minor viral infection. These sorts of illnesses should be treated symptomatically—that is, treat whatever symptoms seem to be bothering the child most.

Although they're not too common, a few more serious infections can include belly pain. Strep throat will almost always include a sore throat and fever, and can often cause abdominal pain, headaches, or vomiting as well. Bellyaches that are accompanied by a high fever and cough may be pneumonia and should be evaluated by your doctor.

Although appendicitis is not common in preschoolers, it can occur at any age. The abdominal pain is severe. Classically, the pain begins near the belly button and a few hours later moves to the lower right side of the belly. However, preschoolers may not clearly describe this sort of picture. In older children and adults, a useful clue is that vomiting begins *after* the abdominal pain of appendicitis. If your child's abdominal pain is so severe that she refuses to move, she needs to be evaluated urgently.

There are many other causes of abdominal pain:

- Urinary tract infections can include abdominal pain, in addition to painful or frequent urination.
- Diabetes can include abdominal pain as an initial symptom of a diabetic crisis, especially if in retrospect your child has been urinating frequently. A simple quick urine test can make sure that neither diabetes nor a urinary infection is present.
- Any of the causes of chronic abdominal pain reviewed later in this chapter can look like acute abdominal pain when they first begin.

ACUTE ABDOMINAL PAIN: WHEN SHOULD PARENTS WORRY?

Three-year-old Tess does not seem well. Last night she started complaining of pain in her belly button, and through the night she's been up a few times vomiting. This morning, she seems even more uncomfortable. She says her tummy hurts "all over" and she's reluctant to stand up straight. When her mother gently squeezes her belly, she winces and pulls away. When they call the pediatrician's office, Tess's parents are told to take her to the emergency room without offering her any breakfast.

A few important clues can distinguish between an emergency-room belly-ache and a bellyache that can wait until tomorrow. Have your child point to a location on the belly where it hurts, using only one finger. If he points right at his belly button, the pain is very unlikely to be anything serious. If he can't point with one finger—that is, if he just sort of pats or rubs his belly all over—then it's also nothing to worry about. The children who need urgent evaluation have specific pain in one point, away from their belly button.

Another useful way to make sure your child's abdominal pain is not an emergency is to see if the belly is tender. Take a gentle squeeze, then push around here and there. Don't ask if it hurts

> ☞ **Mild pain in the belly button is not worrisome, unless it starts moving somewhere else.**

when you do this, but just watch your child's reaction as you squeeze and press. If Junior doesn't flinch and complain, it's unlikely that the bellyache itself is something that should send you immediately to the emergency room. But if your child's belly is tender—that is, painful to touch—you need to get to a doctor quickly.

The most important "red flag" of all is the general appearance of your child. If your child has a bellyache and is still running around, you don't need to

> ☞ **Call your doctor or go to the emergency room if your child's belly is tender to touch.**

worry. If your child is lying on the couch with pain but is willing to sit up, eat a little, and smile, then you might wait a day or so before seeking a medical evaluation. But if your child curls up with pain and isn't willing to get up, you need to head to your doctor's office or an emergency room.

If your child's abdominal pain seems very worrisome—that is, severe, or tender, or accompanied by a high fever or dehydration—you should discuss this with your doctor's office before bringing them in for a routine appointment. Some of these kids will be better served by going straight to the emergency room, where quicker laboratory and radiology services are available. They may need to be sedated for their evaluation, so don't offer anything to eat or drink until after they've been seen.

CHRONIC ABDOMINAL PAIN

Mild infections rarely last longer than two weeks. If your child has long-lasting pain then other causes need to be considered. Two specific causes are reviewed in other chapters: constipation in Chapter 12 and lactose intolerance in Chapter 16.

Many preschoolers have "functional abdominal pain," more formally called "chronic recurrent abdominal pain." (This has an unfortunate acronym that occasionally shows up in a physician's note.) This is abdominal pain that doesn't have a specific medical trigger; even in-depth testing is not going to show any problems. This pain seems to be triggered by overly sensitive nerves in the gut—that is, it occurs in people who find normal abdominal sensations to be painful. In most of us, gas bubbling or stool squeezing around isn't particularly painful, but in some people this sort of normal gut activity is felt as painful. Often, this runs in families. In adults, it's called "irritable bowel syndrome." If one or both parents report that they, too, often have bellyaches it can help explain what's going on with the child. Though there may not be a specific medical cause, the pain itself is real and should not be dismissed. Usually a diagnosis of functional abdominal pain is suggested by the history and physical exam. This can be confirmed with a relatively small number of inexpensive and not-too-invasive tests. If your child has chronic abdominal pain accompanied by "red flags" (see below), more extensive tests will be necessary.

> Belle, age four, is brought to the pediatrician after being picked up from school for the third time this month with bellyaches. She's a happy child, and is in overall good health. There has been no vomiting, no diarrhea, and no weight loss. She says her belly hurts "right in the middle." In the office she is able to comfortably jump up on the table. After asking more questions and doing a careful exam, the pediatrician asks mom to keep a diary of when the pain is occurring. Mom discovered from her notes that Belle's complaints are almost always on the three days a week she attends school, or sometimes during the evening on nights before school. Some open-ended questions about school reveal that Belle has become scared of one particular child she thinks is picking on her.

Although there isn't an exact medical word for it, more common than functional abdominal pain in preschoolers is what I'll call "situational abdominal pain." This is the child that only gets a bellyache on mornings they have to go to school, or in the afternoon right before swimming lessons. Again, I don't think kids this age are "faking it." Their pain is real, and they are really uncomfortable. But what's needed is a little parenting psychology rather than any sort of "medical" intervention. Pay close attention to the pattern and triggers of your child's bellyaches to see if there's a situational trigger. You may want to bring your child to the pediatrician to discuss this sort of pain, as it can be therapeutic and reassuring to the child to have a trusted doctor make sure their belly is okay. For patterns of abdominal pain that are functional or situational, review Chapter 23 for additional tips on how to conduct your own therapeutic discussions with your child.

Gastroesophageal reflux disease (GERD) occurs when stomach contents come up backwards through the esophagus. Though occasional spitting occurs in almost all babies, some children have pain with their spit up. They may twist their head back or sideways, or contort themselves in another shape to prevent reflux. Reflux pain is usually worse after eating. Though we've always thought that most babies with painful reflux outgrow this, a substantial percentage of babies with GERD continue to have painful reflux when they're older. Some of these kids complain of less specific belly pain, though most will have more obvious heartburn symptoms like vomiting, spitting, or a "yucky" taste in the back of the mouth. GERD can run in families, too.

Celiac disease is an intolerance to wheat protein that is far more common than previously thought. It occurs in at least 1 in 200 children. The classic symptoms include poor growth, abdominal pain, and diarrhea; many kids have other symptoms including constipation or abdominal distension. Symptoms outside of the abdomen, such as rashes or behavior problems, can occur with or without the belly complaints. A blood test can be used to look for celiac disease in patients with suggestive symptoms or a suspicious family history.

Rarer causes of abdominal pain in children include peptic ulcers, kidney obstructions, migraines, endocrine disorders, and many others. If your child is suffering from long-running abdominal pain, you may need to work with your pediatrician as well as GI (gastrointestinal) and other specialists for appropriate evaluation and treatment.

Though most cases of chronic abdominal pain can be evaluated with a step-by-step, careful process, some warning signs make it more likely that a serious problem needs an urgent diagnosis:

- Weight loss
- Slowed growth
- Persistent fevers
- Persistent or severe vomiting or diarrhea
- Specific pain located at a single point away from the belly button
- Unexplained or abnormal physical exam findings

EVALUATION

The evaluation begins with a careful history and physical exam. Usually, this is sufficient to get a clear diagnosis. If necessary, the first tests done are usually on urine and stool. A plain x-ray of the belly can be helpful to confirm constipation, but is otherwise rarely helpful. A "barium swallow" or "upper GI series" is often ordered to evaluate reflux, but it cannot confirm or exclude the presence of GERD. It is only helpful to exclude anatomy problems, or perhaps to screen for ulcers. There is no evidence suggesting that blood tests or ultrasounds are likely to help a child who does not have "red flag" findings. More invasive tests occasionally ordered or performed by specialists include endoscopy or CT scans with IV contrast. Keep your own records of all tests, and bring them with you to your pediatrician and any specialists involved in your child's care.

THERAPY

If a specific diagnosis is known, therapy is chosen specifically for that problem. For instance, GERD sufferers take antacids, and kids with strep throat should take antibiotics. Even in children who do not have a specific diagnosis, there are good ways to help abdominal pain feel better.

For mild bellyaches, don't forget how important touch can be. A gentle belly rub followed by a heating pad or hot water bottle can be wonderful. Encourage any child with a bellyache to try to go to the bathroom.

Diet is important. For acute abdominal pain, encourage a blander diet of frequent, smaller meals. If abdominal pain is more long-lasting, a healthy diet includes more water, less juice, more whole grains and fresh fruits and vegetables, and fewer processed foods. You may be tempted to restrict certain foods, thinking they may be triggering pain. If you do this, try not to let your child know, and deliberately rechallenge him with a food that had seemed to cause problems to really confirm that the food is the culprit. Kids with chronic abdominal pain will often have good days and bad days, so don't be too quick to implicate a certain food without doing some confirmatory back-and-forth trials. If your child reliably gets pain every time a certain food is consumed, then stop giving it and discuss the implications with your pediatrician.

Medicines may help:

- *Older antacids (Maalox, Mylanta, Tums, Rolaids, many others)*. These are safe at any age, and quickly reduce the acid in the stomach. Try them especially for upper abdominal pains, using the liquid forms for younger children who cannot use chewables.
- *Middle-age antacids (Zantac [ranitidine], Pepcid [famotidine], others)*. By blocking one of the triggers of acid secretion, these decrease stomach acid for a more prolonged time than the older antacids. The adult versions of these are over-the-counter, though children's liquid forms require a prescription. They have a good long track record of safety and are often tried in children whose abdominal pain is unexplained.
- *Newest antacids (Prevacid [lansoprazole], Prilosec [omeprazole], others)*. The most effective antacids are these newest drugs, which turn off acid secretion in the stomach completely. They can be used with a prescription in children, and appear to be as safe as the other antacids. However, there is less of a track record of safety and none are FDA-approved for use under age one. No liquid versions of these medications are commercially available.
- *Anti-gas medicines (Mylicon [simethecone], others)*. As discussed in Chapter 19, there is no evidence whatsoever that anti-gas medicines are effective in any way. They are safe, and can be used as a placebo to help convince a child that a parent can help.
- *Antispasmodics (Levsin [hyoscyamine], Bentyl [dicyclomine], others)*. Very limited studies show these *might* be effective in relieving abdominal pains in

children. Use them with caution, as there are side effects: sedation, dry mouth, constipation, and confusion are all common.

Overall, the goal of treatment should be to allow the child to return to school and normal activities. It is not reasonable to expect therapy to completely eliminate all pain, and parents and pediatricians should be honest with children about the expectations of treatment. The pain may not disappear entirely, but we can help.

ABDOMINAL PAIN: WHEN TO CALL

! These red flags mean call your doctor now:
- Severe belly pain that prevents walking or standing
- Abdominal tenderness—that is, a belly that hurts to be touched
- Belly pain that hurts worst on the child's lower right side
- A child who is especially ill, uncomfortable, or scared

Bellyaches are common in children, and most of them go away with time and tender loving care. There are some red flags to look out for, but with a careful history and physical examination most children with belly pain can be easily diagnosed by their pediatrician and then managed at home.

12

CONSTIPATION

A regular baby is a happy baby, and constipation is usually easy to diagnose and treat. There are just a few insider tips parents ought to know.

WHAT IS CONSTIPATION?

Children are constipated when they have infrequent, hard, and painful stools. The most important word in the definition is "painful"—if your baby has a bowel movement only once a week, but it's soft and painless, that's not constipation. Likewise, if your baby usually has two bowel movements a day, and then goes three days without the next one, that's not necessarily constipated. Unless the baby is uncomfortable, it's usually best to wait it out.

Pain itself should *always* be treated, whether it's from an impacted wisdom tooth, a broken toe, or from constipation.

> ☞ **If your child's stools are firm but painless, it's not constipation and doesn't need to be treated. The children who need treatment are the ones with painful stools.**

Once your kids are out of diapers, you won't be closely monitoring their stool habits. Suspect constipation if your child complains of abdominal pain during or after meals, or when the pain is located on the child's lower left side. Even children who are having daily stools can become constipated if they aren't emptying their bowels completely.

CAUSES OF CONSTIPATION

Laura is a very active child who runs from one activity to the next. She's become constipated because she just won't sit down long enough to finish completely when she goes to the bathroom.

Hillary is a shy preschooler. She's embarrassed to raise her hand at school, so she holds in her stool all day. Since school started in the fall, she often complains of bellyaches after dinner.

Barbara loves dairy, and often has cheese three times a day plus plenty of milk.

Almost all constipation seen in preschoolers is called "functional," meaning there is no specific medical reason. Sometimes functional constipation runs in families. Diet can also contribute to constipation, especially if a child's intake lacks fiber and water or is overly rich in dairy. However, I don't stress adjusting the diet of constipated children because it can be very frustrating to try to get children to eat differently. Fighting with constipated children to increase fiber intake is likely to make both the parents and child upset, without improving the constipation.

There are some rare medical conditions that can cause constipation. The most serious of these, Hirschprung Disease, begins just after birth with an inability to pass stools. If your child has been "constipated since birth," an evaluation for this condition should be done. Celiac disease, a form of wheat intolerance, can uncommonly cause constipation, as can reactions to milk. A constipated child may also have a rare anatomic or neurologic problem. If your child's constipation doesn't resolve with ordinary treatment, you and your pediatrician should discuss some of these rare possibilities.

PREVENTION AND TREATMENT: NONMEDICAL APPROACHES FIRST

Try to prevent constipation by offering your child an appropriate diet including water, fruits, and vegetables after six months of age. Rely on whole grains rather than processed flour as much as possible.

Even with a great diet, many babies and toddlers suffer from constipation. Help them overcome this issue when it first begins. Early treatment helps children feel comfortable, and also prevents the problem from escalating. Children who have hard stools quickly learn that it hurts to have a bowel move-

> ☞ **Roy's rule #1: Don't be reluctant to treat constipation.**

ment. So they hold it in, which makes the stool even bigger and harder. Untreated constipation leads to a spiral of pain, holding, and worsening constipation.

The key to treating constipation is to find a routine that you can stick to, every day. What you're looking for is the "Goldilocks" stool—not too hard, not too soft, but "just right." If your child tends to be constipated, adjust diet, habits, and medications that are appropriate for your child's age until you find a routine that consistently results in painless stools. Stopping the routine too early can lead to a cycle of ever-recurring hard painful stools. It's better to continue mild therapy every day.

Diet interventions can work with a motivated and willing child. You can try to give juice regularly, especially prune or pear juices that are rich in the natural laxative sorbitol. Most children prefer apple or orange juices, which are not as helpful for constipation. Don't go overboard with the juice—over six to eight ounces a day can contribute to weight problems and dental cavities, and may lead to an overall less healthy diet. Prunes (pureed for babies, or diced for older kids who can chew them) can help with constipation, and are more likely to be accepted if children get used to the flavor when they're young. Consuming more whole grains, fiber, and water can also help children with constipation, *if* they're willing to go along with this plan.

For older kids who are spending time on the potty, daily stooling habits need to be addressed. Kids need to spend enough time on the pot to finish their business—not just to have a two-inch stool and then go back to playing. Encourage children to take their time. Bring a book or video game! Do what it takes to prevent kids from rushing.

Don't attach any negative feelings to stooling behaviors. Make sure that your child doesn't feel "left out" of any fun activities when a break is needed for a bowel movement. Don't send them to the bathroom with a stern command that makes it seem like a punishment. Even subtle cues can lead to trouble. In some families, referring to stool as "stinky" or "yucky" seems to increase the chance that children will become "hiders," ducking behind the drapes or furniture to have a bowel movement in their diapers. Hiders often have trouble with stool holding and delayed training.

MEDICINES FOR CONSTIPATION

Many kids suffer from constipation even with all of the nonmedical issues addressed. For these children, a laxative is necessary.

An ideal laxative tastes good and is easy to give. It should soften stool without causing cramping or gas. It should be very safe and easy to adjust the dose up or down to get a good stool consistency. None of the laxatives commonly used in children are in any way physically addictive, so you don't need to worry about your child becoming "dependent." There are many options, both over-the-counter (OTC) and by prescription (Rx). Speak with your pediatrician before beginning a regular laxative routine to make sure that the safest and most appropriate agent is used.

- *Colace* [docusate sodium] (OTC) is minimally effective, and tastes terrible. There are better options for children.
- *Corn syrup* (OTC as food item) is sometimes added to the formula of infants with constipation. Studies have not shown that it is very effective, but it is safe and may be worth trying.
- *Fiber laxatives* (OTC) include Citrucel, Metamucil, Benefiber, and others. These must always be taken with fluids to prevent constipation, so it's best to use

the ones that have to be mixed in a beverage. Some children may object to the taste or grittiness of the more traditional varieties. If your child will take these consistently, they're safe and effective.

- *Lactulose* (Rx as generic) is effective and safe for any age, and has a nice sweet syrupy taste and consistency. Some kids will develop some gassiness on lactulose, which is available as an inexpensive generic.
- *Milk of Magnesia* (OTC) is very safe and effective, though it is usually not given to babies less than a year or so. It can easily be given in higher or lower doses. Some kids will refuse to take it because of the taste.
- *Mineral oil* (OTC) will work, but should never be taken by babies less than one year. It has no taste but does have an oily consistency that can be hidden in a smoothie-type frozen blender drink. It is very cheap, and is 100 percent effective for children who will take it. Older kids will refuse it when they realize it can cause leakage of oily stool.
- *Miralax* [polyethylene glycol 3350] (OTC) is an excellent alternative. It is a tasteless powder that can be mixed in any beverage, and the dose can be adjusted within a wide range to get daily soft stools. It can be used safely for long periods of time.
- *Senokot* [senna] (OTC) should be avoided. It can cause cramping, and chronic use may damage the colon.

The exact dose of laxative needed will depend on your child, but with experimentation parents should be able to find that perfect dose of medicine to get daily, soft, painless stools. You'll want to stay with that dose long term to establish good habits and avoid painful setbacks.

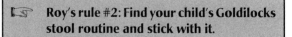

☞ Roy's rule #2: Find your child's Goldilocks stool routine and stick with it.

With careful and consistent use of medical and nonmedical approaches, more aggressive therapies are seldom needed. But if your child is really straining with pain that has not responded to medicines, you may need to use a suppository or enema. Review your long-term care plan with your pediatrician so that use of these types of unpleasant interventions can be

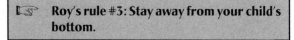

☞ Roy's rule #3: Stay away from your child's bottom.

minimized. It's best to avoid traumatizing children (who are already afraid of their own painful stools) by putting things in their anus.

COMPLICATIONS

Untreated or undertreated constipation can lead to more serious problems. If your child is trying desperately to hold in painful stools, you need to get aggressive with therapy. Use a stool softener to make those stools soft and painless, and keep them soft and painless until your child's memory of the pain is gone.

It may be difficult to tell if a child is holding back a stool, or trying hard to push it out. A sure sign of holding is "the doody dance": dancing and hopping with legs squeezed together.

Children who are constipated are nearly impossible to toilet train. They're just too fearful of their own stools to be willing to have them voluntarily. Treat the constipation first, then move on with the training. If you are training and your child becomes constipated, put all training efforts on hold. While children are training, make sure they can keep their feet flat on the floor or a step stool for leverage. It's more difficult for children to squeeze out a bowel movement with their legs dangling.

Encopresis is a troubling complication of constipation. Children become so used to having a rectum filled with stool that they no longer pay attention to their own body sensations. Their colons become stretched out, and they begin to leak stool around the constipation. Many families refuse to believe that the children don't know what's going on back there, leading to further family tensions, hard feelings, and social isolation. If your child develops encopresis, it needs to be aggressively treated by a pediatrician or gastroenterologist with the experience and temperament to guide a family through long-term therapy to rehabilitate the gut and develop normal stool habits.

Some children with chronic constipation develop bad urinary habits as well. This may be because the full rectum is pressing on the bladder, or from altered nerve signals that begin to occur when a child is so used to being constipated that they no longer get a full sensation when they need to have a bowel movement. These kids may urinate very frequently, wet their beds at night, complain of painful urination, or wet their underpants during the day. When these problems occur with constipation, the constipation must be fixed before any progress can be made with the urinary issues.

CONSTIPATION CAN BE CURED

Keep Roy's rules of constipation in mind:

1. Don't be reluctant to treat constipation.
2. Stick with your Goldilocks routine.
3. Stay away from your child's bottom.

Constipation can make you and your children miserable, and can lead to serious complications. Treat constipation aggressively and consistently to keep your child comfortable and happy.

13

VOMITING

In most cases a vomiting child can be effectively treated with a few simple home care instructions. Parents just need to keep their eyes out for a the red flags that could mean trouble.

CAUSES

Vomiting is usually triggered by a viral infection, often called a "stomach flu" or "tummy bug"—though in fact genuine influenza is very different from an ordinary vomiting illness. Often, the illness will begin with a mild fever and fussiness, especially if the child is too young to complain of nausea. As the illness progresses, vomiting is sometimes followed by abdominal pain and diarrhea. Viruses that trigger vomiting are contagious, so multiple family members can be affected one after the other like dominoes being knocked down. A typical "tummy bug" lasts only a day or two.

Other infections can cause vomiting as well. Bacterial infections of the gut, including Salmonella and *E. coli*, typically cause vomiting along with diarrhea. Many infections outside of the abdomen, such as strep throat and pneumonia, cause vomiting in addition to other symptoms. Although much rarer, diseases of almost any other organ system can include vomiting, from the kidneys and urinary system to the liver, pancreas, or brain. Recurrent vomiting can be a sign of migraine headaches, intestinal obstruction, a block in urine flow, or metabolic diseases. While almost all vomiting is triggered by benign viral illnesses that go away on their own, if your child's vomiting doesn't fit the typical pattern, you'll need a pediatrician's evaluation to ensure that nothing else is going on.

Is It Vomiting or Spitting Up?

Children with vomiting act sick and uncomfortable. They retch, and usually the vomiting has some effort behind it. When babies spit up, they're otherwise happy. The milk comes up without much effort and fuss.

DIAGNOSIS

In a child who has a routine, ordinary vomiting illness, no further testing is necessary to confirm the diagnosis. Sometimes, unusual symptoms in the history or abnormal findings on the physical examination indicate that tests are needed.

Vomiting Plus Other Symptoms: Some Useful Tests

- Severe headache: CT scan of the head
- Vomiting green bile: X-ray of the belly, sometimes after drinking contrast material (sometimes called a barium swallow or upper GI series)
- Bloody diarrhea: Stool examination and testing
- Severe abdominal pain, or pain in the lower right part of the belly: CT scan or ultrasound of the abdomen

Tests can sometimes be useful to tell how dehydrated a child has become, or to look for complications from the loss of fluids. These can include measurements of a child's weight, a urinalysis, and blood tests to look at the body's chemistry and kidney functioning.

TREATMENT

It isn't the vomiting that gets kids in trouble—it's dehydration. When the body loses too much fluid, blood won't be able to reach the brain and other vital organs well. The most important part of therapy for vomiting is preventing and treating dehydration.

Dehydration is best prevented at home with a technique called "oral rehydration therapy," or ORT. This simple and effective therapy has saved millions of lives worldwide. During ORT, the caretaker provides frequent, small sips of appropriate fluids. For infants and younger children, the best fluid to use is a commercially available balanced pediatric electrolyte solution such as Pedialyte. These are sometimes flavored to make them more acceptable (apple is by far the best). Avoid choosing the red flavor—it can look like blood if it is vomited back up. Electrolyte solutions frozen like a popsicle are also available, which prevent kids from gulping the fluid down too quickly. In older children with mild vomiting, a sports drink like Gatorade, mixed to half-strength if the flavor is too strong, is a reasonable alternative. Plain water, juice, and soda are *not* good choices for ORT.

The key to effective ORT is tiny, frequent sips. A good routine for babies or infants is one teaspoon every ten minutes. Don't give them a full bottle and then pull it away—that makes them mad! Instead, put a small volume in the bottle or sippy cup and refill it ten minutes later. When only small volumes are given, vomiting doesn't usually continue; even if the child does vomit again, the balanced electrolyte solution is absorbed quickly to prevent dehydration. Studies have shown that for mild-to-moderate vomiting and dehydration, ORT is more effective than intravenous fluids in preventing complications and long hospital visits. And best of

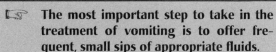

The most important step to take in the treatment of vomiting is to offer frequent, small sips of appropriate fluids.

all, you can do it at home! Be prepared for your child's next bout of vomiting by keeping a suitable rehydration solution handy.

MEDICINES FOR VOMITING

Medicines have a limited place in the treatment of ordinary mild vomiting illnesses; in fact, there are no medicines that are FDA-approved for use in viral-induced vomiting in children under two.

Emetrol. This is a very safe over-the-counter product. It seems especially useful for nausea, though in my experience once a child begins to vomit it doesn't seem to help much. It has a very strong taste, and younger kids may refuse to take it. A usual dose for ages two to twelve years is one to two teaspoon every fifteen minutes. If nausea and vomiting persist for longer than an hour, you should contact your physician for further instructions. Although not FDA-approved, a smaller dose can be given to younger babies. Discuss this with your pediatrician.

Phenergan (promethezine) and *Tigan (trimethobenzamide).* These are two similar prescription medications available in suppositories and other forms to treat nausea and vomiting. The FDA-approved labeling for Phenergan includes a specific warning that it can cause young children to stop breathing, and should never be used for children under age two. Both medicines make children sleepy and disoriented, which makes giving oral rehydration fluids more difficult. These drugs should not routinely be used in vomiting children.

Zofran (ondansetron). Developed to help with the nausea and vomiting that accompanies chemotherapy, Zofran is a newer prescription drug that has shown great promise in limited trials for treating ordinary vomiting in children down to age one. It is being used fairly routinely in many pediatric emergency rooms (ERs), and appears to have very few side effects. However, even the generic form is very expensive. Zofran is available in a melt-in-your-mouth disintegrating tablet.

Vomiting: When to Call

> ! These red flags mean call your doctor now:
> - Vomiting accompanied by severe abdominal pain, especially if the belly is tender to touch
> - Vomiting that occurs in a child that looks quite ill, has a stiff neck, a severe headache, or difficulty breathing
> - Vomiting that is persistent and occurs after a head injury
> - Your child seems especially ill, uncomfortable, or scared

Parents should be aware of the signs of significant dehydration, and seek medical attention if a child develops dehydration and cannot or will not take fluids. Signs of significant dehydration include:

> ! These red flags mean call your doctor now:
> - Urinating less than every four to six hours
> - Sleepiness, lethargy, or listlessness
> - A sunken soft spot on the head in babies less than twelve to fifteen months of age
> - A dry, tacky mouth and lack of tears

Contact your pediatrician during regular hours if:

- Vomiting lasts longer than two days.
- Vomiting is often accompanied by a headache.

Remember it is better to prevent dehydration than to play catch-up once your child has already lost a lot of fluids. Sometimes, dehydrated children will refuse liquids, leaving you no choice but an ER trip. If your child vomits more than once, begin offering small sips of appropriate fluids *before* signs of dehydration develop.

14

DIARRHEA

What's worse than spending the night awake with diarrhea? Spending the night up with your child with diarrhea! The mess, the stink, the crying, and the sheer ick factor have brought parents to tears. Though diarrhea by itself is rarely a cause of serious problems in the developed world, it certainly is a nuisance that everyone would like to avoid. In this chapter we'll explore the insider's world of diarrhea: its prevention and treatment, and how to know when this common annoyance might be making your child more seriously ill.

Almost all of the children with diarrhea evaluated in a pediatric office have what I'll call "ordinary diarrhea." Stools become watery and more frequent, often with some bellyaches or a mild fever. There may be vomiting as well, especially at the beginning of the illness. But ordinary diarrhea is never bloody and should not give your child a fever over 103°F. Children with ordinary diarrhea might seem a little ill, but are never lethargic or unarousable. Contact your doctor for any child who is acting sick or miserable, or for any diarrhea that lasts longer than two weeks. But for ordinary di-

> ☞ **For ordinary diarrhea, there is usually no need to see your pediatrician.**

arrhea in a basically healthy child, follow the suggestions in this chapter before heading to your pediatrician.

CAUSES AND PREVENTION

Most episodes of ordinary diarrhea are caused by viral infections. These illnesses are relatively mild and often begin with a few episodes of vomiting. Occasionally bacterial infections in the gut can cause diarrhea, but even these usually resolve on their own. For diarrhea that lasts longer than two weeks, other causes should be considered, including unusual infections, adverse reactions to food, or conditions that prevent the gut from absorbing nutrition well. In any case, the likely cause of diarrhea can often be determined from the history.

In addition to careful hand washing and other steps reviewed in Chapter 1, there are other important steps you can take to avoid infections that cause both vomiting and diarrhea:

- Wash hands and preparation surfaces well after handling raw meats and poultry.
- Don't keep raw and cooked foods together, and do not put cooked items on a plate that had been holding raw food.
- Don't leave cooked food at room temperature—it should be kept hot or refrigerated.

More information about preventing food-borne illnesses can be found at www.cdc.gov/foodsafety/.

EVALUATION

The evaluation of a child with diarrhea begins with a review of the history. Tell your pediatrician if you've had any foreign travel within the preceding two months, or if there has been contact with other people with diarrhea. Your pediatrician will also want to know how often and how severe the diarrhea has been, and if other symptoms such as vomiting or fever are part of the illness. Try to keep track of how often your child urinates—though it is difficult to know

> ☞ **Don't give anything brightly red to eat or drink to a child with vomiting or diarrhea. That red color can reappear in vomit or stool, causing unnecessary worry about blood.**

when there's urine in a diaper along with diarrhea. The actual color of the diarrhea isn't a very useful detail unless it is blood red.

The most important aspect of the physical exam is the child's overall appearance. An active, bright, and playful child is not seriously dehydrated and needs no special evaluation or therapy for diarrhea other than extra fluids. But if your child appears listless or in pain, you may have a serious problem on your hands.

Laboratory testing requires the parents to collect stool samples, a messy process that is almost always unnecessary. However, more chronic diarrhea might require stool or blood testing to reach a diagnosis. A thorough lab evaluation is warranted for prolonged diarrhea associated with weight loss.

> ☞ **Collecting and testing stools is unnecessary for ordinary diarrhea that lasts less than two weeks.**

TREATMENT

The goal of treating ordinary diarrhea is to prevent dehydration. Offer frequent sips of extra fluids. If you're nursing, nurse more often; for babies younger than six months, a balanced electrolyte solution such as Pedialyte is a good supplement to ordinary formula during diarrhea. For older babies, sips of any fluid are ordinarily fine including water, juice, or sports drinks. If your child has symptoms of dehydration, work with your pediatrician for more precise recommendations on the fluid types and amounts you should be offering.

A child with diarrhea should continue a regular diet. There is no evidence whatsoever that a diet restricted to bland or starchy items helps diarrhea improve—in fact, such a restricted diet is likely to *prolong* diarrhea. The single exception to this may be milk. In some studies, excessive milk consumption has been shown to prolong diarrhea, especially

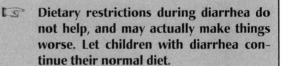

Dietary restrictions during diarrhea do not help, and may actually make things worse. Let children with diarrhea continue their normal diet.

among children from the developing world with more severe illness. For children in the developed world, drinking ordinary amounts of milk or milk-based formula is not a problem.

A few medicines can be useful in the treatment of diarrhea:

- *Imodium (loperimide)* can be used down to age two, and is somewhat helpful for limited use in mild illness. However, it slows down the gut, potentially preventing children from getting the infection out of their bodies. Do not use Imodium for a more serious diarrhea that includes a high fever or bloody stools, or for diarrhea that results from the use of antibiotics.
- *Attapulgite* is a clay-like material that has been touted to "absorb toxins and bacteria." Kaopectate used to be the most commonly available form, but attapulgite was removed from Kaopectate several years ago when it became clear that it really didn't work at all.
- *Pepto-Bismol (bismuth subsalicylate)* may help cramps and diarrhea to some degree. Because it contains an aspirin-like ingredient, doctors are reluctant to suggest Pepto for routine use in children. Aspirin itself has been linked to Reye syndrome, a rare but very serious disorder that in the past had occurred when children with certain viral infections took aspirin. Kaopectate, which used to contain the worthless attapulgite, now contains the potentially dangerous bismuth.
- *Probiotic supplements* include brands such as Culturelle and Lactinex. These contain billions of beneficial live bacteria, similar to the bacteria that turn milk into yogurt. In some excellent studies, ingestion of probiotics helps with some of the more common viral causes of diarrhea. Probiotic supplements are very safe, and are worth a try to help relieve diarrhea in children.

Frequent, watery stools can be rough on a baby's skin. Change diapers as soon as possible after each stool, and allow the skin to dry naked for as long as possible—if you're feeling lucky. Help the skin dry by using a fan or *cool* hair dryer. Apply a thick layer of white diaper paste (zinc oxide, available in Balmex, Desitin, and many others) to protect the skin. If any red diaper rash lasts longer than four days, begin using an anti-yeast cream (such as Lotrimin AF [clotrimazole]) twice each day. If your child's diaper rash is uncomfortable, a soothing medicated ointment containing hydrocortisone 1% (Cortaid) can be added.

The bottom line (sorry) about the treatment of diarrhea is keeping your child well hydrated and comfortable. Medications don't help very much, but fortunately diarrhea usually improves in a few days. Remember that children with diarrhea as well as everyone involved in their care should wash or sanitize their hands frequently.

Children with diarrhea who have free access to fluids will drink more, preventing dehydration. Your child will be at much higher risk for dehydration if vomiting and diarrhea occur together. See Chapter 13 for more about the symptoms and treatment of dehydration in children.

CHRONIC DIARRHEA

Though most episodes of diarrhea last only a week or so, children occasionally develop chronically loose stools. The list of causes of chronic diarrhea is long, but most of these conditions are too rare for most parents to worry about. I'll review two of the most common causes of chronic diarrhea, along with one rarer cause that might fool your doctor.

Toddler's diarrhea is the most common cause, by far, of chronic diarrhea in a preschool child. Typically, this begins at the age of twelve to eighteen months in an otherwise happy child who is growing well and gaining weight as expected. There is no belly pain, and the stools are mushy with bits of undigested food. Toddler's diarrhea arises when the diet is too rich in carbohydrates such as juice, crackers, and bread. If parents are eager to treat toddler's diarrhea, the diet needs to be adjusted to include more protein, more fat, and less juice. Consuming more whole grains rather than processed flour and refined sugar can also help. In an otherwise thriving toddler, it is not really necessary to "treat" this sort of diarrhea unless it is leading to diaper rashes, or the child keeps getting sent home from day care for suspected infectious diarrhea.

Celiac disease is a complex disorder that is triggered in susceptible individuals by exposure to gluten, a protein most commonly found in wheat. Although most physicians were taught that a child with celiac disease would be extremely ill, it is now known that there is a wide spectrum of symptoms in celiac disease.

Some children may be only mildly affected, with mild diarrhea or abdominal distension as the only symptoms. Celiac disease is common, occurring in at least 1 in 200 people, and if left untreated can lead to serious complications including cancer, osteoporosis, and psychiatric problems. It is easy to screen for celiac disease with a simple blood test.

Lactose intolerance deserves special mention because it is misunderstood by physicians and families alike. Though very common in adults and teenagers, true lactose intolerance is very uncommon in the preschool age. Almost everyone is born with a good capacity to digest lactose, which is the main sugar in human breast milk. Lactose intolerance arises later in life, often in the teenage years. Some infant formulas are marketed specifically for lactose-intolerant babies, catering to misinformed families rather than fulfilling a genuine need.

DIARRHEA: WHEN TO CALL

> ! These red flags mean call your doctor now:
>
> - Blood mixed with the diarrhea
> - Severe belly pain
>
> Parents should be aware of the signs of significant dehydration and seek medical attention if a child develops dehydration and cannot or will not take fluids. Signs of significant dehydration include:
>
> - Urinating less than every four to six hours
> - Sleepiness, lethargy, or listlessness
> - A sunken soft spot on the head in babies less than twelve to fifteen months of age
> - A dry, tacky mouth and lack of tears

Contact your pediatrician during regular hours if:

- Diarrhea is accompanied by weight loss or significant pain.

Although diarrhea is common, in the developed world it is usually not serious. Some of the "cures" touted aren't of much help, and may in fact be harmful. If your child has diarrhea, you need to do only a few things: wash your hands frequently, offer extra fluids along with a normal diet, and try to prevent a diaper rash. Seek medical attention for any diarrhea that makes your child act ill with a high fever, dehydration, or bloody stools. You should also take your child to be evaluated by your pediatrician for diarrhea lasting longer than two weeks, especially if there is weight loss. A quick evaluation with a minimal number of tests is usually all that is required to diagnose and treat ordinary diarrhea in children.

15

Environmental Allergies

Allergies to pollen, indoor molds, animals, and other environmental exposures can begin in preschool-aged children. The sneezing, runny noses, and itchy eyes can occur year-round (with house dust or cat allergy), or can be seasonal (with pollens). For most children, these sorts of allergies are more of a nuisance than a serious problem. But in some children the symptoms are severe enough to disrupt sleep and make it difficult to concentrate in school.

WHAT CAUSES ALLERGY?

An allergic reaction is an altered immune response to an otherwise innocent trigger, or "allergen." Our immune systems are supposed to attack and fight off infectious invaders, while ignoring other things our bodies encounter. Sometimes this reaction goes haywire, and an immune response occurs when it isn't needed. Depending on the kind of response, a person might experience a rash, vomiting, difficulty breathing, or nasal and eye symptoms. For the environmental triggers reviewed in this chapter, almost all allergic symptoms are limited to the nose and eyes.

Some families seem to have more allergic problems. Often, environmental allergies appear in the same people or families as asthma, eczema, and food allergies. Together, these disorders are sometimes called the "atopic diseases."

Allergies are becoming more common. For environmental allergies, this may be because our children in the developed world are exposed to far fewer "unclean" challenges. Evidence for this so-called "hygiene hypothesis" shows that without early exposures to ordinary infections that are commonly seen in most of the world, children are more likely to develop allergic diseases. Likewise, some allergic symptoms are seen less often in children who are raised on farms, perhaps because of their exposures to agricultural pollens and animal dander. At this time there is no practical or safe way to expose your child to more illnesses or other allergens in the hope of preventing potential allergic problems, though research involving administration of "probiotics" shows promise.

SYMPTOMS

Environmental allergies most commonly cause symptoms collectively called "hay fever," such as:

- Itchy, pink, and watery eyes
- Itchy nose
- Sneezing
- A watery, drippy, or clogged nose
- Rubbing at the nose
- Coughing from postnasal drip

Though allergies are sometimes blamed for headaches, fatigue, dizziness, or poor school performance, these other symptoms would only occur as a result of the main allergic symptoms. If your child is having these sorts of symptoms without any nose or eye complaints, it is not an allergic problem.

Children with allergies often have a certain "look." Frequent upwards nose rubbing, called an "allergic salute," can leave a shallow horizontal crease in the middle of the nose. There may also be dark or purplish circles under the eyes, called "allergic shiners."

> ☞ **If your child doesn't have nasal or eye symptoms, it's unlikely that environmental allergies are causing any other problems.**

Allergic noses are either "cloggy" or "drippy," depending on whether the lining of the nose is swollen and clogged, or secreting mucus that drips. The distinction is important because these symptoms should be treated differently.

Comparing Typical Symptoms of Allergies Versus the Common Cold

Allergy	Common Cold
Begins with nasal symptoms	Begins with a sore throat
No fever	May have fever
Lots of sneezing	Some sneezing
Some coughing	Lots of coughing, especially near the end
Nasal mucus is watery and clear	Nasal mucus becomes thick and yellow near the end of the illness
Other atopic problems often present (eczema, food allergies, asthma)	Other atopic problems absent
Year-round, or spring and fall	Mostly winter
Eye symptoms common	Eye symptoms uncommon

DIAGNOSIS

Will, age four, has a runny nose and is sneezing a lot. He hasn't had a sore throat or a fever, and no one else in the household is ill. Mom recalls that last year at the same time—in August—he had very similar symptoms that improved with Benadryl.

The diagnosis of environmental allergies is usually made clinically, from the history and physical exam. Sometimes the exact allergic trigger can be ascertained from the child's story. Allergic symptoms that begin in mid August are often triggered by ragweed pollen; or perhaps itchy red eyes only occur when the cat is nearby. Sometimes a more formal history, using a calendar to record the exact timing of symptoms, can be helpful for an allergist to review.

If allergic symptoms are severe or difficult to treat, testing can help identify specific triggers (see Chapter 16). When evaluating environmental allergies, testing can be especially useful in certain circumstances:

- *When allergy symptoms are disruptive and can't be controlled by medications.* In this case, better avoidance may help—but the trigger has to be identified. If avoidance fails, testing can allow a program of immunotherapy (shots) to be designed.
- *The family is considering getting rid of a family pet.* In some cases, a cat or dog can trigger significant allergy. I suggest you have your child tested before getting rid of a pet. Perhaps allergies have nothing to do with Fido or Tabby.
- *Before investing in expensive air filtration equipment.* For some allergies, effective whole-house filtration can decrease exposures and symptoms. But good systems are very expensive. If you are considering installing an expensive system, have your child tested first to see if it is likely to help.

THE PITFALLS OF TESTING

Allergy testing looks for specific triggers chosen from a panel. There is no way to test against all potential triggers, so it is possible your child is allergic to something that wasn't on the test. However, most allergies are caused by only a handful of common triggers, and these are included in the usual panels.

Allergy testing is more reliable to "rule out" than to "rule in" allergy. If your child has a negative allergy test, it is very unlikely that there is a true allergy to any of the tested allergens. However, a positive test doesn't always mean there is a real allergy. To know for sure if a tested positive is really causing symptoms, it is best to perform

> ☞ **A positive allergy test does not always mean your child is allergic, but does indicate that an allergy is likely.**

an "open challenge." Try to stop exposures to see if symptoms stop, then deliberately reexpose the child to see if the symptoms come back.

TREATMENT OF ENVIRONMENTAL ALLERGY

The first step is avoidance of the triggers. This is not always possible—some allergens are common everywhere, and some children have triggers that are difficult to identify. Still, if your child is suffering from allergic symptoms you should at least try some common sense, inexpensive allergen avoidance:

- Keep dust levels down by vacuuming carpets, keeping blinds and fans clean, and limiting the number of stuffed animals in your child's room.
- Don't let pets sleep in your child's bed.
- Use a specially designed cover on mattresses and pillows to reduce dust mite exposure.

Many medications are helpful:

Antihistamines are available over the counter (Benadryl [diphenhydramine], Claritin [loratidine]) or by prescription (Allegra [fexofenadine], Zyrtec [cetirizine]). They relieve sneezing, itching, and nasal drip; they do not help with a clogged nose. They may help with eye symptoms as well. Older medicines like Benadryl need to be taken more frequently and are sedating, which may be fine if they're only needed at nighttime. The newer drugs (Claritin, Allegra, Zyrtec) are less sedating but are not more effective. Because less-sedating Claritin is available over the counter and in an inexpensive generic form (as loratidine), it is the best antihistamine to choose for kids older than two years.

Myths and Facts About Antihistamines

Myth: Antihistamines can help with the common cold.

Fact: They don't help with nasal symptoms, but they are mildly sedating and can help your child sleep.

Myth: People with asthma shouldn't take antihistamines.

Fact: Antihistamines won't do any harm in asthma. You may have heard that antihistamines somehow "dry up" mucus, making it more sticky. In the past this was feared to be a problem for asthmatics, but this isn't true. The warning label was removed from the most common antihistamine in 1992.

Decongestants (pseudoephedrine or phenylephrine) are available in a variety of over-the-counter or prescription products, often combined with an antihistamine. These can help temporarily with nasal clogging and drip, though using decongestants regularly will decrease their effectiveness. Their best role is for occasional use on very bad days, typically only in children older than two.

Steroid nasal sprays are available by prescription only (Flonase [fluticasone-generic available], Rhinocort [budesonide], many others). These are safe for use in young children, and are the most effective treatment for nasal clogging.

They don't work as quickly as oral medicines, and are best used as a daily regimen during allergy season.

Eyedrops can help itchy and watery eyes quickly and effectively. Try a non-medicated, soothing moisturizing drop first. These are inexpensive and give quick, temporary relief (they work even better if refrigerated). The older and inexpensive over-the-counter medicated eyedrops work (Opcon [naphazoline], Visine [tetrahydrozoline], and others), but they tend to sting and sometimes cause rebound symptoms. Zaditor (ketotifen) changed from prescription to over-the-counter status in 2007. It's very effective and comfortable, though expensive. The best prescription choices are Patanol (olopatadine 0.1%) or the newer, brand-only version Pataday (olopatadine 0.2%) which claims to last a full twenty-four hours.

As with all medications, take these products as directed and purchase inexpensive generics when available.

Nonallergic Chronic Eosinophilic Rhinitis

Some children have symptoms that appear to be entirely allergic, with a typical chronically runny or clogged nose. However, they test negative even on extensive allergy panels. Some of these children may have "nonallergic chronic eosinophilic rhinitis," a long-winded way of saying "allergic illness without an allergy." Though a specific allergy can't be demonstrated in these kids, their symptoms improve markedly with inhaled nasal steroids. They do not benefit from antihistamines.

IMMUNOTHERAPY

For those whose allergy symptoms are severe and don't improve with medical therapy, immunotherapy can provide relief. In immunotherapy, specific allergy triggers are identified and given in very small doses in a series of shots. The exact program may vary, but in general shots are given frequently at first (perhaps once a week), tailing off to perhaps every other month within a few years. In some cases, undergoing a whole course of immunotherapy permanently eradicates the allergy.

Immunotherapy is rarely used in preschoolers, whose allergic triggers may not yet be "set in stone." These young kids also have so much fear of needles that ongoing immunotherapy can truly be miserable. There is always a risk of a severe allergic reaction being triggered by immunotherapy injections, so allergy shots should only be administered in a facility that can respond to an emergency. Kids undergoing allergy shots must wait for observation at their doctor's office after each injection. However, even with the hassle and risk, immunotherapy is an important last resort that has helped many people overcome their allergies.

Some practitioners, especially those outside of the United States, administer immunotherapy by placing material on or under the tongue. Though ongoing research may make "sublingual" immunotherapy a good option in the future, for now this has not been established as effective and is rejected by the majority of American board certified allergists and their professional societies.

Bee Sting Allergy

A very serious environmental allergy can be triggered by the stings of bees, wasps, fire ants, or other insects. In children who have these allergies, life-threatening symptoms can begin very quickly: difficulty breathing, swelling of the throat, vomiting, widespread hives, and unconsciousness. If your child has experienced these sorts of symptoms you should work with an allergist to confirm the trigger and consider immunotherapy so that your child is protected. You should also have a device to inject epinephrine available at all times.

Reactions close to the sting are not too worrisome. That is, if your child is stung on the hand and his arm swells up, this is not considered a serious reaction (you should still treat the sting with Benadryl, cool wraps, and painkillers). However, if that same sting on the hand leads to symptoms of the airway or chest, or if your child develops a widespread rash, contact your doctor or call 911 right away.

Environmental allergies to pollens, dust, animals, or molds are common in children and adults, often beginning before school age. Try some basic avoidance strategies and safe medical therapy without visiting a doctor. For more severe or difficult-to-treat symptoms, visit with your pediatrician or an allergist for guidance on the best prevention and treatment strategies.

16

FOOD ALLERGIES AND SENSITIVITIES

If you read food labels, you might start to think that food allergies are common and very dangerous. After all, your breakfast cereal might have been manufactured in a facility that also processes peanuts! Surely, if they went through the trouble of putting that phrase on a label, it must mean something. Right?

Though most adverse reactions to food are not serious, life-threatening reactions can occur. Understanding the difference between potentially dangerous allergic reactions and more mild problems can help you avoid food anxieties while still protecting your child from genuinely dangerous exposures.

TRUE FOOD ALLERGIES

Though many doctors lump all adverse reactions to foods as "allergies," this oversimplifies the wide range of reactions that are seen. It is important to know whether your child has a true allergy or a different kind of food sensitivity, so you know what to expect and how vigilant you need to be about food safety.

True allergic reactions to food can be serious. In these reactions, food-specific antibodies, called "IgE," are created that trigger a potentially massive immune response should they ever come in contact with their food target. It is as if a child's immune system has mistakenly decided to attack a food item as a foreign invader. The food that triggers the reaction is called an "allergen."

At his two-year birthday party, Luke was eating some cookies with peanuts. Ten minutes later, he developed raised, red, splotchy areas first on his face then on the rest of his body. He started coughing, and his voice sounded squeaky and soft. His parents did the right thing: they stopped him from eating any more cookies, and called for an ambulance.

The symptoms of these classic food allergies can vary from person to person, and can even be different upon repeated exposures. They can begin within seconds of an allergen exposure, and almost always begin within a few hours. Skin reactions are the most common reactions, appearing as hives. These are raised, warm, red, itchy areas that appear suddenly on many areas of the body. Individual hives clear on their own within several hours, but new hives can continue to develop. Sometimes hives are accompanied by swelling of the face, lips, or tongue, called "angioedema." Other symptoms of true allergy can occur in the gastrointestinal (GI) tract, including vomiting and stomach cramps. Diarrhea

☞ **Some food reactions can become more serious with repeated exposures: hives, vomiting, and breathing difficulties. If your child has had these symptoms, it is very important to avoid future exposures.**

that occurs very soon after an exposure may be a true allergy. Serious respiratory complaints can also occur, such as swelling of the tongue and throat, wheezing, and difficulty breathing. More rarely, a serious allergic reaction can cause a drop in blood pressure, unconsciousness, and death. Any child who has had any of these kinds of reactions is at risk for the most serious manifestations of food allergies upon exposure to their trigger food.

The most common foods to trigger true allergic reactions in children are milk, peanuts, tree nuts, eggs, soy, wheat, shellfish, and fish. You may be able to prevent the development of some of these allergies by delaying introducing these foods to your child, especially if you have a family history of food allergy. Speak with your pediatrician to find out the best strategy to avoid exposures while still offering a nutritious diet to your child. It is especially important for mothers who come from families with food allergies to nurse their babies rather than rely on milk- or soy-based formulas.

The best "treatment" for allergic reactions is to avoid exposures. If you know your child is allergic to a food item, learn to study food labels to look for hidden sources of the food. One good Web resource for parents is www.foodallergy.org, a nonprofit organization whose Web site includes information about food labels and allergen avoidance. In true allergies, even small exposures can trigger reactions. If your child attends group care, you may need to make sure that no sharing occurs between the kids' lunches. Though it is possible for an extremely allergic individual to react to minute traces of a food in the air, for almost all allergic kids it's only necessary to make sure they don't eat the food.

Though avoiding exposures is the most important step, be prepared to treat an allergic reaction if one does occur. Parents of allergic kids should always have Benadryl or another antihistamine handy, and use that immediately for any hive-like reaction. For any more serious reaction, including any difficulty breathing or decreased consciousness, an injection of epinephrine should be given without hesitation.

Allergies to most food items are usually outgrown over a few years. This includes milk, egg, wheat, and probably most other foods. It had been thought in the past that peanut, tree nut, fish, and shellfish allergies are lifelong, though even these can eventually be outgrown in some children. Work with your pediatrician or an allergist to safely find out if your child has outgrown food allergies. It is possible for children to not always react; just because your child safely ate eggs once doesn't mean the allergy is gone. Allergic manifestations may or may not occur every single time an allergic child is exposed.

Who Should Carry Epinephrine?

Epinephrine (sometimes called "adrenaline") can be lifesaving. It can reverse the progression of even the most serious allergic reactions almost instantly. It must be given by injection. Parents can use an automatic device with a spring-loaded needle (one brand name is "Epipen"). But which parents should carry one of these devices all of the time?

Certainly, any child with a history of life-threatening allergic reactions should always have epinephrine available. Also, certain foods are more prone to cause severe reactions than others. The scariest offender is peanut, so many allergists recommend that anyone with peanut allergy should keep epinephrine close at hand. Another clue to the potential for a severe reaction is the presence of asthma. Almost all children who die of life-threatening allergic reactions to foods have a history of recurrent wheezing, or asthma.

If your child has asthma *plus* food allergies, is allergic to peanuts, or has ever had a life-threatening reaction to any food, you should have injectable epinephrine available near the child at home and at school, all of the time.

Benadryl (diphenhydramine) plays an important role in the therapy of true allergic reactions. It doesn't act as quickly as epinephrine, so it shouldn't be given alone in a true emergency. For hives without any other symptoms it is reasonable to give only Benadryl and watch the child closely. If your child has had hives as part of an allergic reaction, keep Benadryl handy.

As mentioned earlier, many packages of food contain warnings about items being processed on equipment that touched nuts, or in a facility that uses milk. These labels are meant to prevent lawsuits, and really aren't helpful. For most families with food-allergic children, avoiding foods that actually *contain* the allergen is important; avoiding foods that may have come *near* the allergen is silly. Furthermore, these lawyer-written labels may lead to a tremendous amount of anxiety and a diet that's limited, unappealing, and inadequate.

Are Hives Always Caused by Food Allergies?

No. In fact, a child with a first episode of hives who has no obvious recent unusual food exposure is much more likely to have hives triggered by a viral infection than by a food. Most of the time in clinical practice, the history of a food triggering hives is apparent from the initial presentation: "He had salmon, and ten minutes later developed hives." Sometimes, repeated cycles of exposures leading to hives can lead to a diagnostic clue. If your child has *recurrent* hives, a food diary is the best diagnostic tool. Even in children with recurrent hives there is not always a food allergy trigger.

OTHER FOOD REACTIONS

Contact Dermatitis and the Oral Sensitivity Syndrome

Some kids will develop only a local rash on their face, on the area near the mouth that touched the food. The rash can be impressive and itchy. Fortunately, this kind of reaction does not worsen or cause problems elsewhere in the body. Kids with this kind of limited "contact" reaction to certain foods should avoid the food itself, but do not have to worry about more severe reactions.

Sometimes, reactions only occur from the skin of a fruit. Some kids get a rash when they eat whole apples, but are fine if their apple slices are peeled.

Though the biologic mechanism is different, some children complain of uncomfortable oral sensations such as tingling or burning after certain foods, especially apples, mangoes, cherries, and celery. Many of these children happen to be allergic to ragweed or other pollens, too. Though this so-called oral sensitivity syndrome doesn't become more serious, it can be difficult to know if a young child complaining of oral sensations has mild itching or a swelling throat. For this reason, any oral symptom in a child should be taken seriously and assumed to be a true allergy.

Eczema

Eczema is a chronic, scaly, itchy rash that can affect children of any age. For more about identifying and treating eczema, see Chapter 18.

The cause of eczema is controversial. Allergists feel that most eczema is triggered by specific food allergies; if these can be identified and avoided, the eczema will improve. Dermatologists are convinced that most eczema isn't related to any food exposure, and treat the rash with topical moisturizers and medicines.

In truth, it can be very difficult to identify a specific food trigger in most children with eczema. This may be because there are a variety of foods that act as triggers, and that the rash can begin several days after the food exposure. Many very common foods can be triggers, including wheat, egg, and milk—and these are very difficult to avoid.

From a practical point of view, most mild-to-moderate eczema is best treated with the dermatology approach: take care of the skin with moisturizers and medications. If eczema is particularly bad or hard to control, focused testing and challenging can sometimes help identify at least some of the triggers. But don't go overboard. Sometimes parents become convinced that a very long list of food items is to blame, and their children are allowed to eat so few foods that they suffer nutritionally.

Bloody Stools

Some babies develop mucusy and bloody stools beginning at one or two months of age. These babies are almost always fed milk-based formula, and have developed a sensitivity to milk protein. This is sometimes seen in soy-fed babies, and very rarely in babies who are nursed (presumably from milk proteins in mom's diet).

Babies who are fed milk-based formula and develop bloody stools should be switched to another formula, usually a hypoallergenic product such as Alimentum or Nutramigen. Though some of these babies will do well on soy-based formula (which is far cheaper), about half of them will continue to have bloody stools unless a truly hypoallergenic formula is used. For nursing babies, talk with your pediatrician about steps that may include restrictions in mom's diet.

Milk-protein sensitivity usually appears in a mild form, with blood in stools in an otherwise well-appearing and growing baby. This is called "proctitis," and is almost always outgrown by the time a baby is one year old. By then, the babies can begin taking whole milk and dairy products without problems. However, it is important to avoid dairy in these babies until they've reached age one to avoid continued gut inflammation and sensitization. Rarely, milk-protein sensitivity can be more severe, causing poor growth, vomiting, and diarrhea in addition to the bloody stools.

Lactose Intolerance

The main sugar in all mammals' milk (cows and humans) is lactose, which requires a specific enzyme to digest. Almost all human babies have plenty of this enzyme at birth, and keep it for many years. In some people, especially those of African or Asian descent, the ability to digest lactose decreases with age. That's why many teenagers and young adults develop abdominal pain, bloating, and gas after consuming dairy products.

But even if both parents are lactose-intolerant, their baby will almost certainly be able to digest mother's milk or a milk-based formula. Do not worry about lactose intolerance in your baby, and don't waste your money on lactose-reduced formulas.

If your older child develops symptoms suggestive of lactose intolerance, do a simple open study: Choose a Saturday and give your child plenty of milk. If the child is lactose-intolerant, every time milk is consumed symptoms will occur. Though uncomfortable, lactose intolerance does not lead to more serious reactions.

Nasal Congestion

Nasal congestion, drip, or stuffiness is certainly a symptom of environmental allergies to things like pollen or animal dander. These symptoms, reviewed in more detail in Chapter 15, can also accompany other allergic reactions to foods, such as hives. But it is very uncommon for foods to trigger nasal congestion in children who have no other symptoms of food allergy.

Does milk cause nasal congestion? It's doubtful. Though you may sense a sort of stickiness or an unctuous mouth feel when consuming rich liquids such as milk, this isn't mucus. It's perfectly fine for kids with congested noses to continue to consume milk.

Behavior Changes

Can specific foods cause behavior problems in children? Good controlled studies (where parents, children, and independent observers do not know what a child has eaten) have consistently failed to show that items like sugar, high fructose corn syrup, or additives really change behavior in kids. Still, it makes good sense to try to reduce the consumption of processed sugars for the overall health of your children. A diet high in processed food does increase a child's risk for other health problems, including obesity, diabetes, and dental problems.

ALLERGY TESTING

True allergies are caused by a child's own immune system reacting to an otherwise innocent food trigger. Though far from perfect, allergy testing can be a helpful guide as long as you understand its limitations.

Allergy testing can be done directly on the skin of a child, or on a specimen of blood. In skin testing, a small amount of the potential allergen is scratched into the skin to see if a hive appears. The bigger the hive, the greater the chance that the child is truly allergic. Skin testing can only test against a limited number of potential allergens, especially in younger kids who don't have as much skin to use for testing. It is also possible for serious reactions to occur, caused by the small amount of allergen in the test pricks. Both false negatives and false positives can also occur. That is, sometimes kids react on their skin to a food to which they're not allergic, and sometimes a skin test can be negative despite the child having a true allergy. The exact accuracy of allergy testing depends on the skills and methods of the testing center, as well as the kind of allergens being tested.

Blood tests for allergy can be easier to do, as they don't require repeated pricks on the skin of a squirming toddler. They also eliminate any risk of triggering an allergic reaction during the test. The current most-reliable method of blood testing is called a "CAP-RAST." Blood tests can still give you false positive results (that is, the blood test predicts an allergy when in truth there isn't one), but usually if the blood test is negative you can be confident that no true allergy exists to the tested food.

Skin prick testing and CAP-RAST testing can only predict true, classic food allergies. They may or may not be able to predict which children with eczema have food allergy triggers, and are not useful for the evaluation of lactose intolerance, behavior issues, abdominal pain, or bloody stools.

The best "gold standard" test for food allergies is a "double blind placebo-controlled food challenge." Based on the child's history and perhaps test results, foods that are considered as possible triggers are hidden so that the child, parents, and doctors don't know when they are consumed. If the child doesn't react when the food is hidden, an "open challenge" can be undertaken, allowing the child to have a small amount of the food item. Only a repeated identical reaction upon hidden challenge to a certain food really establishes that a child is truly having a reaction.

> ☞ **A positive skin prick or blood test result doesn't always mean your child has a real allergy. A child isn't truly allergic unless real symptoms occur with exposures.**

If your child has had a serious reaction, work with your doctor to determine if testing or an open or blinded challenge is appropriate. You may be asked to give your child a challenge of the food at the allergist's or pediatrician's office, so appropriate medicines and personnel are available in case a reaction does occur.

With more mild reactions, you should try to challenge and rechallenge a child with a food to see if it really is a trigger. We know that most children and adults who *think* they're allergic to foods have no true allergies when tested in this manner.

Older types of food allergy testing can include IgG and IgG$_4$ tests, which often yield multiple "positive" results that do not predict true allergy. Other tests for food allergy have no valid basis and are used by quacks and charlatans. These include sublingual tests, tests of lymphocyte activation, kinesiology, and electrodermal testing. Many families have been misled by these procedures, and end up relying on expensive supplements and nutritionally inadequate diets. Steer clear of anyone who proposes allergy tests beyond well-established mainstream testing methods.

ALLERGIES: WHEN TO CALL

> ! If your child has signs of a serious reaction, call emergency
> medical services (911) immediately.
>
> - Difficulty breathing or speaking
> - Swelling of the mouth, lips, or tongue
> - Difficulty staying awake

If you suspect your child has had an adverse reaction to a food, review
the history with your pediatrician to see if further challenges or testing is
appropriate. Most children who are thought to have allergies in fact do not,
and most food restrictions are unnecessary and may be harmful to growth and
nutrition. When a genuine food allergy is present, avoid that food and have
an action plan in place to follow after any accidental exposure.

17

Drug Allergies and Adverse Reactions

Medicines are powerful agents. They can help eradicate infections or change the way a child behaves, and can effectively treat surgical pain, nausea, and migraine headaches. Some are powerful enough to kill cancer cells. But all medicines come with a price: they can cause problems, some of which are impossible to predict. Sometimes drugs are used in combinations, which further increase a patient's risk of unexpected trouble. Every parent should be aware of the different ways medicines can cause adverse reactions and how to minimize your child's risk of these problems.

Different Kinds of Reactions Have a Different Prognosis

Any time a medicine causes a problem it is called an "adverse reaction." This is a broad term that could mean just about anything. A pill catching in the throat, or a medicine causing sedation that makes it unsafe to drive, or a child getting a red blotchy rash after penicillin—these are all examples of adverse reactions. To keep things clear, it is useful to separate truly allergic reactions from other kinds of medicine misadventures.

A true allergy to a medicine will only cause a few different symptoms. The most common truly allergic reaction is a rash called hives, which most doctors call "urticaria." Hives are raised, warm, itchy pink areas that do not stay present in one location for more than twelve hours. A more serious allergic reaction called anaphylaxis can occur along with or without a rash. Symptoms of anaphylaxis include difficulty breathing, wheezing, problems speaking, or a drop in blood pressure leading to unconsciousness. Hives and anaphylaxis are also called "immediate hypersensitivity reactions" or "Type I reactions." Unlike other adverse reactions, these allergic reactions can recur or worsen with repeated exposures. If your child has had one of these true allergic reactions to drug, it is best to completely avoid that medicine and any medicines that are chemically similar to it.

Most adverse drug reactions are *not* allergic. In fact, among adults who have had an "allergy" to penicillin, less than 10 percent will have another reaction upon subsequent exposure. The most common drug reactions include flat pink rashes, vomiting, and diarrhea; none of these are allergic in nature. If your child has had a reaction that is not clearly allergic, it makes sense to try taking that medicine again, especially once your child is old enough to talk and describe potential symptoms.

It's important to determine if an adverse reaction is truly allergic. Many children have had a mild rash with amoxicillin. The family has been told it was an allergic reaction, and they're unnecessarily frightened of taking this useful and inexpensive medicine in the future. An unwarranted avoidance of some medicines leads to anxiety and an overuse of less appropriate agents.

> ☞ **Drug *reactions* are common; drug *allergies* are rare.**

PREDICTING ADVERSE REACTIONS

Many medicines have known side effects, such as sedation and dry mouth caused by over-the-counter antihistamines. You can find out about the likely side effects of a medicine by looking at the box, bottle, or the package insert. Unfortunately, the list of adverse reactions that appears in a package insert may be tremendous. Even infrequent reactions are listed individually, and it's difficult to know which reactions are the most important. When a medicine is prescribed for your child, ask your pediatrician about the side effects that are most likely to occur.

Other adverse reactions are difficult to predict. Neither allergic nor nonallergic adverse reactions run in families, so knowing that mom is allergic to an antibiotic does not increase her child's chance of problems. Sometimes individual children can have sensitivities to medicines that might apply to similar medications. For instance, a child who gets hyperactive on one decongestant may well get hyperactive on a different decongestant. Since multiple brand names of cold medicines contain the same ingredients, you'll need to read labels carefully. Learn both the brand and generic names of any medicines that have caused problems for your child.

Sometimes it is not clear whether an allergic reaction has occurred, and it may be difficult to know how to proceed safely. If there are other suitable choices, it may be fine to avoid the potential troublemaking agent, at least until your child is older. Review the exact circumstances of any potential reaction with your pediatrician to help decide what medications, if any, need to be avoided.

PREVENTION AND CROSS-REACTIVITY

Avoid taking unnecessary medications, especially antibiotics, and try to avoid taking multiple medications together. "Polypharmacy" is a term used mostly among physicians treating adults to describe a patient on a long list of medications. These patients have a dramatically increased risk of problems from their medicines.

There are times when an allergy to a certain drug can lead to cross-reactivity. This occurs when a certain drug is so similar to another one that allergies to one increase the risk of allergies to the other. Many physicians and pharmacists are not aware of how our knowledge about potential cross-reacting drugs has changed. For instance, you may have been advised if your child is allergic to penicillin that all cephalosporin antibiotics should be avoided. This is incorrect and leads to unnecessary worry and confusion.

Below is a listing of oral antibiotics that really are potentially cross-reactive, meaning that allergy to one agent might increase the risk of allergy to another. This list only applies to true allergic reactions. If your child has had a nonallergic, less serious reaction to one of these medicines, then a different medicine in that group can safely be tried.

- *The sulfa drugs*: Bactrim (trimethoprim/sulfamethoxazole, also called Septra), Gantrisin (sulfisoxazole), and any other antibiotic whose generic name includes the prefix "sulfa" should all be avoided if there is a history of a true allergic reaction to any of them.
- *The penicillins*: Penicillin, amoxicillin, and Augmentin (amoxicillin/clavulanate) are most commonly used in pediatrics. This group includes any drug with a generic name that includes "-cillin." Avoid all penicillins if your child has had a true allergic reaction to one of these.
- Amoxicillin, Ceclor (cefaclor), Keflex (cephalexin), Duricef (cefadroxil), and Cefzil (cefprozil) all share similar structures. There is a small chance of cross-reactivity to any of these if your child is allergic to one of them. However, the chance of a cross-reaction is small—less than 10 percent—and the risk may be justified if the reaction is mild and your child is old enough to tell you about any troublesome symptoms.
- Two other cephalosporins, Omnicef (cefdinir) and Suprax (cefixime), are similar only to each other. A serious allergy to either of these means the other one should be avoided.

TREATMENT OF ALLERGIC REACTIONS

If your child has signs of a serious reaction, contact emergency medical services immediately (usually by dialing 911).

> ! These red flags are signs of a serious reaction requiring immediate medical attention:
>
> - Difficulty breathing or speaking
> - Swelling of the mouth, lips, or tongue
> - Difficulty staying awake

For most adverse reactions, home treatment is the first step. Stop taking the medication that seems to have led to the reaction, and call your doctor's office to discuss how to proceed. Depending on the circumstances, the doctor may call in a different drug or ask you to rechallenge the child with the first medication.

Give oral Benadryl (diphenhydramine) for any reaction that includes hives. Families should keep Benadryl on hand for unexpected allergic reactions to medications, bee stings, or other reactions. If your child has a raised, itchy rash, you can give Benadryl even before you call the doctor. A single oral dose will not do any harm.

STEERING CLEAR OF ADVERSE DRUG REACTIONS

Follow these insider tips to minimize the chance that an adverse reaction to medication will harm your child:

1. Avoid medicines if they're not needed.
2. Choose the safest medicine that suits your needs. These are often the older, generic products with the longest track record.
3. Avoid taking multiple medications together.
4. Keep track of adverse reactions that affect your child. Make sure you and your pediatrician have an accurate account of any adverse reactions, both allergic and nonallergic.
5. Don't assume that all reactions are allergic.
6. Don't unnecessarily avoid medicines that in the past were thought to have potential for cross-reactions.
7. Remember that almost all adverse reactions to medication are mild and non-allergic.
8. Most reactions stop when the offending medication is discontinued.

18

RASH DECISIONS

Every good pediatrician should be a good dermatologist—and in fact most parents can become pretty good dermatologists, too! Rashes in children almost always fall into one of just a few categories, and often similar treatments can be used for similar rashes. Most rashes are entirely benign. Unless there are certain red flags, parents can usually treat rashes at home for at least a few days before seeking a doctor's opinion.

IS THIS A RASH I NEED TO WORRY ABOUT?

There are only two questions you'll need to ask yourself to help decide if your child needs an immediate medical evaluation for a rash.

First, how is the child doing? If your child's rash is accompanied by other symptoms—listlessness, difficulty breathing, pain, or a high fever—contact your physician right away for instructions. If your child has a rash but is otherwise acting just fine, it is unlikely that you have a serious problem on your hands.

Second, make sure that the rash isn't the kind that can herald serious illness even in an otherwise well child. This worrisome rash, called *petechiae*, looks like little dots of blood under the skin. Sometimes these little dots can group together forming large bruised-looking areas. If your child has a red dotty sort of rash, stretch the skin from either side. If it disappears with pressure, it is not petechiae, and you can be less worried. But a red dotty rash that does not disappear when stretched can be a sign of a serious problem. Call your pediatrician.

The remainder of this chapter reviews the most common rashes encountered in babies and preschoolers: what they look like, how to confirm the diagnosis, and initial treatments that you can start at home. As long as your child is acting well and the rash isn't petechial, you can safely try to diagnose and begin treatment on your own. If you don't see improvement, or if you remain worried for any reason, go see your pediatrician during normal hours.

You can call first, but rashes are very difficult to diagnose over the phone—your doctor will probably want to see it rather than guess.

ALLERGIC CONTACT DERMATITIS

This is an allergic reaction in the skin, limited to the area that touched the trigger. It's very itchy and red, and sometimes scaly. Common triggers include:

Poison ivy, oak, and sumac. Look for raised blisters along with itchy streaks of red bumps. Often the rash is worst on the thin skin near the face and occurs in streaks and lines where the plant touched the skin.

Nickel. You may see areas of inflamed skin where the backs of clothing rivets and metal clasps touch skin.

Shampoos, conditioners, detangling sprays, fabric softeners, and detergents. You'll find itchy red areas near the scalp or in areas where clothing bunches up.

To begin treatment, try to identify and eliminate the cause. If you've switched to a new fabric softener, go back to one with fewer chemicals and fragrances. If the rash seems related to metal clasps, get rid of those clothes or paint the metal with clear nail polish. If a rash begins after a day in the woods, give your child a good bath and clean up any clothes and other items that could still be contaminated with sap or plant oils.

After further exposures have been prevented, treat the rash itself. A cold, wet hand towel (leave it in the refrigerator) wrapped around an itchy area feels great. You can also try an anti-itch colloidal oatmeal bath. Topical medicines include calamine or over-the-counter hydrocortisone. Oral Benadryl (diphenhydramine) can help the itching too, but don't bother with topical Benadryl. When applied directly on the skin, Benadryl can actually cause the child to develop an allergy to the medicine! If the allergic contact dermatitis is severe, visit your pediatrician for more instructions. A more potent topical or oral steroid might be needed.

ECZEMA

Eczema is a common, chronic, itchy rash of childhood. It can begin in infants, and though it usually goes away in a few years, it can occasionally persist through adulthood. The rash can be anywhere, but often prefers the creases of the elbows and knees. In babies, it's most prominent on the cheeks. Eczema is red, scaly, and *always* itchy.

There are plenty of things you can do to help with eczema:

Keep the skin well hydrated. In winter, use a humidifier to prevent dry air from worsening eczema. Avoid letting your child soak in soapy water. Instead, allow children to play in the tub *before* adding the soap. When it's time for washing, use a mild soap and quickly rinse off. Immediately after every bath, apply a heavy coat of a thick moisturizing cream to already-wet skin.

ALAMEDA FREE LIBRARY

Treat itching. You can use over-the-counter oral Benadryl, or a prescription such as Atarax (hydroxyzine). Cool moist wraps can help, too. You want to keep the itching under control; scratching will make the rash worse and keep everyone up at night.

Treat the skin inflammation. Most of the medicines used to treat eczema are topical steroids. They work well and are very safe if used properly. Ointments are less irritating and more effective than creams. Hydrocortisone 1% is available over the counter, and might help with the mildest eczema, but often a stronger prescription product is needed. Newer eczema medicines include the nonsteroid creams Protopic (tacrolimus) and Elidel (pimecrolimus). Though these were quite popular when introduced, use of them has dropped off since warnings became publicized about their being linked to cancer. The warnings apply only to long-term use on large body areas, but many physicians have steered away from these newer drugs.

Eczema is in the family of "atopic" or allergic-type diseases, which also include asthma and allergic rhinitis (hay fever). If your child's eczema does not improve with simple therapy, consider looking for a possible food trigger. See Chapter 16 for more details about the possible relationship between eczema and foods. With careful dietary avoidance, about 15 percent of children with eczema can have a food trigger identified.

Eczema should be managed as a daily problem—that is, even when the skin is looking good, you should continue with your daily moisturizing regimen. Occasional flare-ups can then be more easily controlled with low-potency medications. Eczema can usually be managed by you and your pediatrician, but if your child's eczema is failing to improve with your pediatrician's advice, ask for a referral to a dermatologist.

HIVES

Also called urticaria, hives are raised, pink, warm areas of skin that can occur anywhere on the body. Individual hives themselves will always move, shift, and change over a few hours. A good trick is to circle a hive or two, and recheck in twelve hours. If the spot didn't move, it isn't a hive. Hives may be of nearly any size, from little pinheads to big blobby areas. If they're big, sometimes the center of the hive begins to clear up before the edges, so it can look like a big irregular raised circle.

Although hives in adults are usually triggered by a specific exposure, usually a food allergen, in children this is not the case. Most hives in kids are triggered by mild viral or bacterial infections with minimal other symptoms.

Hives are best treated with an oral antihistamine such as Benadryl. Double-check the dose with your physician, as we will often use a higher dose than is listed on the package to treat hives. Benadryl wears off in about six hours, so be prepared to repeat the dose. Newer antihistamines do last longer, but don't seem as effective in treating hives. In a serious emergency, pediatricians trust Benadryl. Typically, antihistamines are continued for a few days after the rash is gone.

INFECTIOUS RASHES

Rashes in children are often triggered by infections. Sometimes, other symptoms and features of the infection are the best clues; other times, the rash itself is so characteristic that a good look from an experienced parent, teacher, or health care worker yields the diagnosis. In this section I've only included the most common infectious rashes you're likely to see.

Chicken Pox

Routine vaccination against chicken pox, also called "varicella," has made this rash infrequent. Breakthrough cases that occur in vaccinated kids are milder, with few lesions and little fever. The classic chicken pox that many parents remember isn't seen much anymore: a day of fever followed by five days of crops of itchy skin spots. The spots start as red bumps that develop into blisters, which pop open and crust over. Because new crops of pox erupt over several days, you can see both old and new lesions on the same child. The incubation period for chicken pox is ten to twenty-one days.

Children at high risk for developing severe chicken pox include infants less than one year of age and those with poor immune systems. Adults are also prone to severe chicken pox if they are not immune from vaccination or childhood exposure.

If your child has chicken pox, keep the lesions clean with routine baths. Treat the fever with Tylenol (acetaminophen), and treat the itching with topical calamine, cool wraps, an oatmeal bath, or oral Benadryl. Contact your physician if your child is miserable or has new or worsening fevers after four days. Also contact your pediatrician if you have an unimmunized child at high risk for complications who has been exposed to chicken pox.

Fifth Disease

Triggered by a viral infection, Fifth Disease includes a very characteristic rash: the cheeks look red as if they've been slapped, and the outside surfaces of the arms and legs develop a lacy, flat pink rash. Most children lack any other symptoms, though older girls and adults will sometimes have joint aches and other problems. Fifth Disease can trigger serious complications in women during the beginning of pregnancy, or in people who have problems with their red blood cells. As long as your child and her contacts are not at special risk, Fifth Disease requires no treatment or isolation.

Hand-foot-and-mouth Disease

This viral infection is usually seen in summer or early fall. Though called hand-foot-and-mouth disease, the rash may not be in all of these places. Most of the rash may occur on the legs, buttocks, or other areas. The rash itself may be nondescript, with little raised red dots, or may include classic small white oval ulcers on a red base. Spots in the back of the mouth tend to be painful and may prevent your baby from wanting to eat or drink. The rash on the body is usually painless. Often children will run fevers during the illness.

The main therapy for Hand, Foot, and Mouth Disease is to continuously offer cool, soothing liquids to prevent dehydration. Ibuprofen or acetaminophen can be used for fever. Sometimes, topical agents are prescribed to numb the spots in the mouth.

Impetigo

Impetigo is a superficial skin infection, usually with staph or strep bacteria. It starts with an area of skin that is injured—say, by a scrape or insect bite. Then bacteria from the environment invade and cause the area to turn pink with a yellow or shiny crust. Sometimes cloudy blisters are present. Once bacteria have colonized an area of impetigo, it is easy to spread to other parts of your child (or other children) through scratching.

When your child has impetigo, try to keep the area clean. Gently scrub the area with ordinary soap and water at least once a day. In most circumstances, ordinary (not antibacterial) soap is fine, though sometimes a medicinal soap such as chlorhexidine is suggested. Areas of impetigo should be kept loosely covered to prevent spread to other children.

For mild, small areas of impetigo, use a topical over-the-counter antibiotic ointment (Polysporin, bacitracin, and many others) three times a day until the rash heals. More extensive impetigo will need a prescription antibiotic cream (Bactroban [mupirocin]; others) or an oral antibiotic. In most parts of the United States, the best oral antibiotic for impetigo caused by staph is Bactrim. Before starting oral antibiotics, it is best to take a swab of the area for culture to confirm which bacteria is present and which antibiotics will treat it best.

If impetigo is recurrent, your doctor may suggest other ways to decrease bacterial colonization. This can include longer courses of oral antibiotics, special soaps, or adding a small amount of bleach to the bathwater (about one-fourth cup of household bleach per bathtub).

Other Viral Exanthems

Many other viral infections can trigger rashes, and typically tests are not done to confirm exactly what the trigger is. These rashes, also called "exanthems," are usually flat or minimally raised, and do not itch. They don't move around like hives, and are often concentrated on the trunk and back—though they may appear anywhere. If your child has a rash along with a low-grade fever or other viral symptoms, it's probably triggered by a mild virus that requires no therapy.

Roseola

Roseola is a specific viral rash that follows a very characteristic course. A baby will have three days of fever—sometimes quite high, up to 105°F. The fever responds well to medicine and in fact when the fever comes down the baby seems quite well. After three days, the fever ends. Then, a subtle flat pink rash begins on the back before spreading to the rest of the body.

Typically, the rash and the time course of the infection are so characteristic that no tests are needed. Sometimes, though, the high fever leads to an evaluation with blood and urine tests to make sure there is nothing more serious going on. Once the rash appears, the diagnosis is easy. Roseola itself requires no treatment beyond supportive care for the fevers.

Scarlet Fever (Scarletina)

Scarlet fever is a red, raised, sandpapery-feeling rash that arises during a strep infection. The rash is most noticeable on areas where the skin is pressed by clothing, such as right under the beltline. In years past, the strep organism was more virulent and good antibiotics weren't available. The infection is now easy to identify and treat, so the rash is often called by a different name—scarletina—so we don't scare the grandparents.

INSECT BITES

They itch, and they're usually limited to exposed skin. Though fleas only bite adults on the lower legs, children are shorter and can get bitten anywhere. Mosquitoes are probably the most common insect biter, and are much more active in the summer. Be especially wary of being outside right at dusk, when mosquitoes are actively looking for their next meal.

Try to prevent insect bites by eliminating their sources. Pets can be dipped for fleas, and mosquitoes will be less common around your home if you eliminate their breeding spaces in areas of standing water. If your kids get bitten a lot, consider calling an exterminator to safely cut down the insect population. Use insect repellant sprays containing the active ingredients DEET or picaridin. These are safe and effective when used as directed on children. There are many herbal alternatives to repellants, but the only ones that work reliably are products containing "oil of lemon eucalyptus."

Treat insect bites by keeping them clean to prevent infection. Topical steroids like hydrocortisone (over-the-counter) or more potent topical prescriptions can be very helpful, especially if applied as soon as possible after a bite. Oral Benadryl will also help with the itching and swelling that accompany bug bites.

NEWBORN RASHES

Many newborns develop rashes, and almost all of these are harmless. They'll disappear without treatment. As with other rashes, you should be more concerned if your newborn has a rash and is acting ill. Call your doctor right away for *any* newborn with a fever or poor feeding. For more information about rashes and other "newborn normals," see Chapter 20.

One special and worrisome rash in newborns is skin that has blisters. This can be caused by herpes simplex infections, which can be disastrous for newborns. If your newborn develops any sort of blistery rash, contact your pediatrician and get evaluated quickly.

SEBORRHEA

Seborrhea is a waxy, scaly, not-itchy rash that's mostly seen in the scalp, neck, and behind the ears. Sometimes it can also occur in the diaper area. On the scalp, seborrhea is called "cradle cap" in babies and "dandruff" in adults. Although it may look unappealing, seborrhea isn't itchy and doesn't make hair fall out.

Treatment can include scrubbing at the scales with a sudsy washcloth, or picking out the scales with a baby comb. You can also loosen the scales with dandruff shampoo, but that can burn your baby's eyes. More severe cases can be treated with topical antifungal products (including Nizoral [ketoconazole] shampoo) or topical steroids such as hydrocortisone.

WARTS AND MOLLUSCA

Common warts and molluscum contagiosum (often called "mollusca" for short) are both annoying skin lesions that are difficult to treat. Though they are triggered by two different viral infections, I've lumped them together in this section because they're unlike other infectious rashes.

Warts are most commonly found on the hands or feet, but they can occur anywhere. They usually poke out of the skin and have a lumpy appearance. Mollusca also occur anywhere, often in small groups, and look like waxy domes with a tiny dent in the center. Neither warts nor mollusca cause symptoms, and in fact they will go away on their own in young children if you just let them be. But it may take years for them to resolve, so many parents seek treatment. Keep in mind that these are not serious problems, and ordinarily don't bother the child. Stay away from any therapy that's painful or dangerous.

Available therapies for warts or mollusca:

Cantherone (also called cantharidin or blister beetle juice) is applied at the doctor's office and can make the lesions red and blistery after a few days. After blistering, they should fall off. Cantherone is less useful for larger lesions.

Curettage is a fancy word for scraping lesions off. This does work, but is painful. If your doctor wants to do this, ask that a topical anesthetic cream be used first.

Duct tape can be effectively used to get rid of warts. In one study, the "duct tape method" was more effective than dermatologist's liquid nitrogen application. The duct tape method involves gently scuffing the top of the wart with a pumice stone or emery board, and then covering the wart with duct tape. The next day, the duct tape is removed and the steps are repeated. Later studies have failed to confirm the effectiveness of the duct tape method, but it is safe, painless, and easy to try.

Liquid nitrogen, applied by a dermatologist, freezes the wart or mollusca. Treatment hurts the next day.

Oral medications, including griseofulvin (an antifungal medicine) or cimetidine (also called Tagamet, an ulcer medicine), work at least sometimes for the eradication of these bumps. We really aren't sure why they work, but it may have to do with altering the body's immune system so the warts or mollusca are recognized and attacked.

A *potato* can be used as part of one colorful way to get rid of these things. In "the potato method," the child has to pick out a perfect potato at the supermarket, and then cut it in half. After rubbing the wart or mollusca with the cut half potato, the child buries it in the backyard. Believe it or not, this method seems to be about as effective as anything else you can try. It's painless and fun, and might just work! Consider the potato method, especially if it helps your child feel that she's in charge of the cure. It might at least help you put off a more painful option.

Salicylates (including over-the-counter Compound W, and many others) are applied once a day, slowly wearing down the lesion. These products are commonly used for the home treatment of larger warts in particular, but with a careful steady hand you can use them to dot small warts. To avoid pain and irritation, avoid getting these products on the healthy skin surrounding the warts.

All of these individually work about 60–70 percent of the time; if one fails, try another. Some physicians combine multiple methods, say by applying a salicylate underneath the duct tape or by applying Cantherone after liquid nitrogen. It seems that every pediatrician and dermatologist has their own favorite way of attacking these nuisance lesions, and because no one method is nearly 100 percent effective, a variety of tricks are tried.

> **Warts and mollusca aren't serious, even if they are a little ugly. Try painless things first.**

Rashes: When to Call

> ! These red flags mean contact your doctor now:
> - A child with a rash who is acting ill
> - A rash that looks like little red dots under the skin, and doesn't disappear when you stretch it

Contact your pediatrician during regular hours for a routine appointment to evaluate any rash that is bothering you or your child.

Dermatology is fun—you can see exactly what you're treating and how it responds to therapy. Many rashes are mild and resolve on their own, but if your child is acting sick or has a worrisome rash, visit your pediatrician for an accurate diagnosis and appropriate treatment plan.

19

THE FUSSY NEWBORN

Newborns are tough on parents. Sleep is one big issue—babies don't sleep when they're supposed to, and parents barely sleep at all. Often, parents are worried about their eating, too. Are they getting enough? Is the milk upsetting them? Are they having normal stools? But by far the biggest concern about little newborns is their crying. They cry too much, and sometimes it's difficult to know why they're crying at all. Fortunately, most newborn crying has an ordinary explanation, and there are good ways to help soothe newborns and give parents a rest.

In this chapter, when I say newborn I mean babies less than three months old. If your baby was born prematurely, the "newborn" period may last longer—you can add that three months to your child's due date, rather than their birth date, to get the approximate date that they'll graduate from the newborn fussy period.

How much crying really is too much? There's no exact answer. For some families, quite a bit of crying is tolerated before anyone worries; for others, fifteen minutes of crying might be overwhelming. The amount of crying that exceeds "normal" depends on the parents, their support system, their expectations, and their level of fatigue. As a pediatrician, the definition I use for "too much crying" is crying that is going on long enough to worry the parents. If the parents are upset, then I'd like to help them out.

For babies, crying doesn't necessarily mean pain. They don't really know any words, so anything they try to say comes out as "waaaaaa!" We also know that pain medicine, like acetaminophen (Tylenol), doesn't consistently help babies who cry excessively. Most newborn crying is not because of pain.

I'm going to divide the causes and cures for crying into two kinds: the quick fixes and the usual suspects. The quick fixes are just that—easy to diagnose, quick to cure. After you've made sure none of these quick fixes apply, you should go into "soothe-the-baby" mode. But if your baby is often fussy without any quick fix reason, then it may be time to think about some frequently seen causes of the persistently fussy baby. These "usual suspects" are common, easy to treat causes of ongoing newborn fussiness.

If your baby is fussy in a way that doesn't fit into these categories, contact your pediatrician right away. You should be especially quick to call your pediatrician if your baby is acting very differently than usual, or if fussiness is accompanied by other problems such as vomiting, fever, pale skin, or any other symptom that you find worrisome.

THE QUICK FIXES

There are only five in this list, and you should be able to tick them off quickly to ensure that they're not the cause of your newborn's crying:

1. *I'm hungry.* If it's been more than an hour or so, try to feed Junior again. You also want to keep an eye on your baby's overall growth and weight. If you have a fussy newborn who is not gaining weight well, by far the most likely cause is hunger. Babies really do go through growth spurts—periods of a few days now and then when they're much hungrier than usual. You can't time the growth spurts, so don't expect a calendar to tell you when to expect them. Growth spurt fussiness is more exaggerated in exclusively breast-fed infants, because they can't quickly get more milk produced. For nursing moms, the way to get through a growth spurt is to feed more frequently.
2. *I'm cold.* Babies whose feet, hands, and foreheads are cool should be bundled up.
3. *I'm hot.* Babies who feel warm (or sweaty if they're more than a month old) may need to be unbundled. Babies less than three months old should always have their temperature measured with a thermometer if they feel warm. Contact your pediatrician immediately for any newborn measured rectal temperature over 100.4°F.
4. *I'm wet.* Some babies hate a messy diaper. Beware the stealth poop—newborn stools might not warn you with much of a smell. If your baby is fussing and has a messy diaper, change it.
5. *My foot is caught up in my sleeper.* When little ones get their foot or arm caught up, they can't free themselves. Help them get untangled if they're upset.

When your baby is crying, go through these five items quickly in your mind. You ought to think to yourself something like this: "She just ate . . . she isn't cold, she isn't warm . . . diaper is fine . . . and her feet aren't tangled up . . . OK, time to soothe the baby."

HOW TO SOOTHE A NEWBORN

Even if there isn't a quick-fix problem, your baby still needs some help settling down. Going from upset to happy isn't an automatic skill, and for the first few months most babies need a little guidance to learn how to settle down. There are some excellent methods to try:

Bundle your baby. Newborns like to feel snug and secure. They may struggle at first, but once they know they're secure, they often settle right down. You should have the nursery staff, a good midwife, a doula, or an experienced nurse or pediatrician teach you how to bundle up your baby safe and tight. Some parents like to use special blankets that make bundling easier. One I've used can be purchased through www.miracleblanket.com.

Hold your baby. Use a gentle hold, with a little bit of a rock. Don't swing them around.

Try a pacifier. Babies find sucking very soothing, and it isn't fair to expect mom to be able to nurse constantly. There's good evidence that pacifier use while sleeping can decrease the chance of Sudden Infant Death Syndrome (SIDS). But if you really just don't like the idea of a pacifier, don't use it.

Try white noise. You can buy a white noise generator at about any baby store or specialty electronics retailer. Choose one that can run on batteries for when you're pacing around with your baby; plug it into an outlet for overnight use. Get your baby used to settling down for naps and bedtime by turning on the white noise and continue using it through the night as an excellent sleeping cue. Turn up the volume to drown out ordinary household noises.

Put your baby down. You'll be surprised: sometimes after all of the pacing and rocking, babies just want a little time of their own. In any case, you probably deserve a rest. There is no reason for anyone to feel that they should always hold their crying baby. Take a rest now and then. Even if your baby keeps yelling, the break will do you both good.

You may be tempted to put your baby down on her tummy to see if that decreases the fussiness. But we know that making sure your baby is put down to sleep on her back reduces her risk of SIDS by half. Also, babies who usually sleep on their backs seem to be especially at risk for SIDS if they are put down on their tummies to sleep.

THE USUAL SUSPECTS

Why do some babies cry more than others? A few common reasons account for almost all of the fussier newborns. By watching their pattern closely and discussing these with your pediatrician, you'll probably be able to quickly determine the cause of your baby's fussing.

Usual Suspect #1: Colic

Marissa, now five weeks old, has always been a bit fussy. She's fine as long as she's held or bundled, but gets upset when her diaper is changed or when she's first put down. Lately, though, every evening has been a nightmare. From 6:30 to 9:00, she yells nonstop. She doesn't seem to be hungry, and can only be soothed for a few minutes before starting to cry again. Her dad is especially unhappy about this— she seems to start her crying spell the minute he gets home!

Almost all newborns will fuss more in the evenings. This reaches its peak when babies are about six weeks old, and goes away entirely by three months of life. For many babies, you could set a clock by it—the baby will cry from say 8:15 to 9:45, every single night.

Why do they do it? Who knows. It isn't really pain, because pain medicine doesn't help. We also know that babies with colic are not in fact any more likely to have more gas in their tummies. By the obvious fixed timing of colic, we know that it couldn't possibly be a food allergy, or anything that mom ate. If it were something in the diet, then the baby would be fussy all of the time. To me, the most reasonable explanation of colic is that it is a period of "blowing off steam" at the end of a day that must seem quite overwhelming to a baby.

What to do for colic? Try the soothing methods above, or try putting Junior in a car seat next to the clothes dryer. Go for a long drive. Be sure to trade places with another adult now and then so that everyone gets a break. Rarely, medicine can be used to provide some respite. Remember: colic goes away at three months!

Usual Suspect #2: Temperament

Some babies are kind of touchy and easily set off. If their arm waves around on the changing table, they get scared. They find the sensation of gas bubbling around in their bellies upsetting. If you've got this sort of baby, concentrate on the soothing methods listed above. Bundle extra tight, and rely on a white noise device to drown out upsetting sounds. Fortunately, babies with a tough temperament improve with time, though they may always be a little slow to warm up to new things. Give your baby hugs and reassurance, and try not to let your own anxiety upset your baby more. If you find that consistently using soothing methods keeps your baby happier and calmer, then use them until your baby learns to be more secure and comfortable with the outside world. This will happen sooner if you're cool, calm, and confident.

Usual Suspect #3: Food

Although not as frequently as many people think, some babies do have trouble with tolerating certain foods. This is far more common in bottle-fed babies. If your bottle-fed child is consistently fussy throughout the day, and soothing doesn't help, talk to your pediatrician about a change in formula. It is easy enough to try a soy product, or one of the inexpensive "easy digesting" formulas such as Carnation Good Start or Enfamil Gentlease Lipil. (These formulas are made by partially "predigesting"—breaking down—some of the proteins. This is supposed to make them easier for babies to digest.) Very rarely, a truly hypoallergenic formula with fully broken down proteins such as Alimentum or Nutramigen is necessary for babies who cannot tolerate ordinary formula, but I wouldn't rush to try these. They are expensive and usually unnecessary.

Some formulas touted as fussiness reducers are a waste of money or unsafe for your baby. The lactose-reduced formulas make no sense, as lactose intolerance almost never occurs in newborns. (Lactose is the natural sugar in mother's as well as cow's milk.) The more sinister formula types that should also be avoided are the ones packaged as "low-iron." Like the lactose-reduced formulas, the low-iron products exist only to take advantage of the fears of parents. No study has ever shown that low-iron formulas are beneficial for fussiness, and we do know that dietary iron is absolutely essential for a baby's health and development. In fact, because the formula manufacturers know that iron is essential, low-iron formulas have been quietly redesigned to increase their iron content. There is no reason to use lactose-reduced or low-iron formulas in the diet of any newborn.

> Cody is three weeks old, and his mother is worried that something in his diet is making him fussy. He nurses well, but seems to be in pain for about fifteen minutes after every feeding. Mom already tried eliminating milk from her diet, which didn't seem to help. At the pediatrician's suggestion, mom decided to stop nursing for three days, offering Cody only a hypoallergenic formula. During those three days, Cody's fussiness continued, confirming that the diet wasn't a problem. Mom resumed nursing and enjoying her normal diet. Cody's fussiness seemed to improve when his family concentrated on soothing techniques rather than worrying about mom's diet.

For nursing babies, it may be difficult to know for sure if anything in mom's diet could be contributing to fussiness. In one recent study, nursing mothers who restricted the nuts, fish, wheat, egg, and dairy products from their diets didn't feel that their babies had any reduced crying. And a restricted diet can be a burden—moms may find it difficult to get the nutrition they need, and they may resent not being able to have foods that they enjoy. Mothers of newborns have enough to worry about, so I do not like to add to their woes and guilt by pushing changes in their own diets. Nonetheless, if a certain meal does seem to consistently lead to fussiness in a baby, it makes sense to try some targeted temporary diet changes to see if that helps. One other approach is to put a nursing baby on a hypoallergenic formula for three days while mom pumps. If during those three days a dramatic decrease in fussing is seen, then perhaps a dietary angle needs to be explored. But if the baby's temperament doesn't change, nursing can be resumed without further worry about diet.

Usual Suspect #4: Reflux

All babies spit up. They have no idea how big their tummies are, so they'll occasionally take a few extra gulps that have to come back up. If your baby is perfectly happy while spitting up, reflux is not a problem.

Other babies have pain with spitting. They cry right after meals, or arch their backs, or squirm around unhappily for a few minutes before a burp. These babies are said to have "gastroesophageal reflux disease," or GERD. If your baby is fussy and has GERD symptoms, talk to your pediatrician about these and other treatment options:

- Slow down the feeds and pause for frequent burps. Unfortunately, this makes some babies even more angry. They may cry, gulp more air, and spit up more. This strategy isn't for everyone.
- Keep babies upright during and immediately after feeds. But it is not reasonable to ask parents to keep their baby upright for an hour!
- Thicken the feeds (if using a bottle) by adding rice cereal. This may reduce the amount of spitting up, but may not reduce the crying much.
- If bottle-feeding, try a formula designed to decrease spitting. One is Enfamil AR, which uses a modified rice starch that thickens in the stomach.
- Rarely, GERD can be a symptom of formula intolerance, so some pediatricians may recommend a trial of a hypoallergenic formula.
- Medicines may help. Zantac (ranitidine) and Prilosec (omeprazole) are among many medications that reduce acid in the stomach. The babies may still spit, but the medicine should reduce any acid-related pain.

Not a Usual Suspect: Gas

I know this goes against what many pediatricians and grandmothers say, but here's a secret that every parent of a newborn needs to know: gas isn't a source of pain.

I know, I know. Everyone blames fussiness on "gas." But think about it, really. Gas bubbles gurgling around and pooting out really don't hurt. It may scare the child, especially a baby with a touchy temperament, but it really doesn't cause pain. If your baby seems distressed by gassy feelings, hold the baby, hug the baby, and reassure the baby. One hundred percent of the babies I have ever seen with persistent "gas pains" are getting their cues from their parents. In other words, it's the parents' worry about the gas that keeps the babies upset. When your baby passes gas, the best thing to do is to make a little joke. Say, "You sound like your daddy!" and hug your baby with a warm smile. Soon enough, babies will learn to laugh at their own noises. Later on, you might want to teach Junior some nicer habits! As a newborn's parent, your goal should be to teach your child to be unconcerned about normal body sensations. Don't think about gas as something bad to be eradicated, but as something normal to learn to live with.

☞ **Farts don't hurt.**

What about gas medicine, like simethecone (Mylicon)? It's a detergent that breaks bigger bubbles into smaller bubbles—in fact you could wash dishes with it. Supposedly, having more little bubbles rather than fewer larger bubbles is a good thing. It is completely inert and harmless to give to your baby, but you should know that it is entirely a placebo. No good study has ever shown that gas drops help babies feel better. Calm reassurance is the best "medicine" for gas.

MEDICINES FOR FUSSY BABIES

I rarely prescribe any medications for fussy babies, but a few are used:

Alcohol. Many cultures include rituals to give a small amount of brandy or wine to a baby. A few drops on a baby's tongue couldn't really hurt, but I wouldn't suggest it. Besides acting as a sedative, alcohol can lower blood sugar and cause seizures. An occasional glass of wine or beer for a nursing mom will not harm the baby.

Paregoric. This form of liquid morphine was a popular remedy some years ago. It will work—a sleeping baby isn't a crying baby—but narcotics should not be used in a baby who isn't in pain.

Levsin (hyoscyamine). Levsin is marketed as an "antispasmodic," but in fact helps reduce crying by acting as a sedative. It should be used sparingly and with caution, but can provide a respite for families at the end of their rope.

All newborns fuss to some degree and the crying can wear down an already exhausted parent. Most crying has nothing to do with pain, but is rather a baby's way of communicating. Try the tips in this chapter to diagnose and treat most of the common crying of newborns. If your baby has an unusual or frightening pattern of crying, or if you're just plain worried, call your pediatrician.

20

Beyond Fussing: More Newborn Normals

Newborns must feel like strangers in our world. For as long as they could possibly remember, they've lived in darkness, accompanied by the constant sound of mom's rushing blood. Suspended upside down and underwater, for the last few months they've been barely able to move. Then, suddenly, there's light, and sound, and coldness, and air. For the first time they can feel their own bodies from the inside and the outside. They must breathe, eat, and poop. Inside, their circulation and plumbing is changing: rather than pumping almost all of their blood through the placenta to get oxygen, suddenly the blood must go through lungs that have never touched air before. It must be very weird and very new.

During this time of change and upheaval, newborns do a lot of strange things. They breathe funny—sometimes congested and irregular. Their hands and feet can turn blue, and they get upset when their tummies rumble. Their skin can be peely or yellow, and sometimes peculiar rashes appear. All of this—and more—can be absolutely normal in an ordinary newborn baby.

Parents of newborns have a tough time, too. They're exhausted, and mom may be in pain. Sometimes, innocent comments and questions from relatives and friends increase anxiety. Newborns seem weak and helpless and insecure, and some parents feel the same way. And a newborn can tell when their parents are anxious and stressed—and that makes the babies cry and fuss more!

To help parents of newborns feel more confident and secure, I like to review the "newborn normals," peculiar but normal things that are seen in ordinary healthy newborns. Parents may be too exhausted to even ask about some of these funny things, but a quick explanation and reassurance can go a long way toward helping everyone get through this rough time.

Keep in mind that for all of these normals, I'm talking about otherwise healthy babies who were born at or near term, after thirty-seven weeks. For babies born prematurely or with other health issues, you should speak directly to your pediatrician about your concerns. In fact, if you just feel anxious, you should speak with your pediatrician even if you've got a healthy term newborn. The items in this chapter are meant for general reassurance, but don't feel reluctant to look to your pediatrician for more specific information about your individual child.

BLUE EXTREMITIES

Newborn babies have a powerful ability to "clamp down" their blood vessels. Strong rings of muscle around blood vessels that are close to the skin can constrict and limit blood flow, and this ability is much stronger in a newborn than in a baby just a few months older. When these blood vessels clamp down, your baby's hands and feet can look blue or purple. Fortunately, this doesn't harm the baby one bit. There is plenty of blood flow to the foot, it's just arriving from deeper blood vessels that you cannot see.

Sometimes, the blue color occurs when babies get too cool. Warm up blue feet with booties and socks. Cool, blue hands can be tucked at the baby's side in a nice warming bundle.

! These red flags mean call your doctor:

- Blue color around the lips that lasts for more than a few moments
- Babies with blue, cool extremities that do not warm up with bundling
- Babies with a blue color to their body, arms, or legs
- Babies who have blue hands or feet that are feeding poorly, running a fever, or are not active

---

CONGESTION

Newborns have tiny little noses, and even a small speck of mucus can make a big racket. Also, they really haven't figured out how to sniff or blow their nose, so whatever mucus they've got in their little nose is likely to stay there and rattle around.

If your baby sounds like she has a stuffy or congested nose, help her along with a few drops of nasal saline. You could also use a soft rubber bulb to help suck out the mucus. Have a nurse at your pediatrician's office or in the nursery show you how to help "unstuff" a baby's nose.

! These red flags mean call your doctor:

- Congestion that makes it difficult for a baby to nurse or take a bottle.
- Congestion that makes it difficult to breathe. Look to see if ribs are showing, the head is bobbing, or if your baby otherwise seems to be struggling.
- Congestion that is "constant" should be evaluated in person during regular hours.

CRYING

All babies cry. After all, that's the only thing they know how to say! The world is a very new and peculiar place to them. Sensations that are normal to you and I can be weird and scary to a newborn. They may also be hungry, cold, warm, wet, or just fidgety and upset. Chapter 19 covers more details about helping babies who cry excessively.

! These red flags mean call your doctor:

- Crying that occurs throughout the day and night
- Crying accompanied by poor feeding or color
- Crying that seems very different from your baby's usual pattern

---

FUNNY STOOLS

You might not realize it, but adults and children rely on trillions of bacteria living in their large intestines to make a nice normal stool. When babies are born, their guts have no bacteria at all, so their stools are very different from those of older kids. They're runny, they're colorful, and they can be either very frequent or infrequent, depending on the age of the baby.

Normal newborn stools have a consistency somewhere between applesauce and toothpaste. True newborn diarrhea is looser—as loose as water, and it soaks into the gel of a disposable diaper. If your newborn's runny stools sit in a puddle in the diaper and don't soak in, it's not diarrhea. Newborn stools are considered constipated if they're too firm to pass easily and painlessly.

The first stools after birth are called meconium. They're black or very dark green, tarry, and sticky. Within five days the meconium will wash out, and you'll see a more ordinary newborn stool. The color can be anywhere along a wonderful rainbow, from brown to yellow to green, or anywhere in between. This color can change from day to day, and doesn't mean anything important.

A newborn should pass his first stool in the first day of life, and once nursing is established, will usually have at least a small "splash" of stool several times a day. By the time babies are six weeks old, they'll often have far less frequent stools, particularly if they're nursing. A nursing baby can go several days without any bowel movement at all. As long as your baby is happy and active and doesn't have a distended or swollen belly, don't worry about infrequent stools in a breast-fed baby older than a month.

What about the straining and faces that some babies make when they're passing stools? It turns out that having a bowel movement is yet another novel experience for newborns, and they sometimes make a big show out of it. When passing stool, you have to push down with your abdominal muscles at the same time you relax your anus. You might think this is easy and automatic, but many newborns get mixed up and squeeze their buttocks tight just when they're supposed to relax. So instead of having a calm, stress-free passage of stool they squeeze and squeeze and turn red until there's a little explosion of poop. If your baby is getting red-faced and upset when she's trying to poop, help her relax with a gentle hold and calmly rock her legs back and forth in a bicycle motion. She'll get the hang of it!

! These red flags mean call your doctor:

- Stools that are truly constipated—hard and pellet-like
- A firm, tender, or discolored belly
- Stools that remain black past five days of life, stools that are blood-red, or stools that are white or light tan in color

---

Gas

Fussiness, crying, and gas are all reviewed in more detail in Chapter 19. Remember that passing gas, burping, and a rumbling tummy are all a normal part of being human. And none of these really causes *pain*.

Even though gas doesn't cause pain, it can certainly make little babies upset. Those funny sensations feel so different that babies don't know what to do about them, and many get worried and anxious. The best way to help your baby feel better is calm reassurance. Hold your baby, rock, coo, and explain to her that everything is okay. Soon enough, she won't get upset at gas anymore.

! These red flags mean call your doctor:

- Constant crying.
- Crying that interferes with eating.
- If you're worried, visit your pediatrician. Worried parents have worried babies, and that makes gas seem more scary. Sometimes firsthand, personal reassurance is the best medicine for "gas."

Head Shape

When babies are born, the bones in their heads are not fused together. Skull bones can slip and overlap each other to allow safe passage out of the birth canal. After a long labor, many newborns have odd, cone-shaped heads. Not to worry, they'll get rounder soon!

Sometimes there can be bleeding under the scalp. Called a "cephalohematoma," this blood collection can feel squishy and can grow quite large. Most commonly you'll feel one of these above and behind a baby's ear. These heal fine with no treatment, but often a prominence on the skull can be felt even after several months.

Newborns can also have a round swelling right in the center of their scalp. These also heal fine. If a vacuum extractor was used, this kind of swelling can be especially prominent, but it is still not a problem for the baby.

Babies who are temperamentally less active and who spend a lot of time flat on their backs will sometimes get a flattening on the back of their heads. This is entirely cosmetic and rarely needs treatment. To prevent this flattening, have your baby spend some time on his belly while awake and play with him in a variety of positions. At bedtime, vary the positioning of his head by turning him with his head at different ends of the crib.

! None of these are emergencies, but certain "red flags" mean that it is more likely that treatment will be needed:

- A newborn whose head bumps from birth are increasing in size, or whose head is not returning to a round shape after several days
- A baby who is developing flattening of the head, who doesn't seem to be able to move her neck equally to both sides
- Head flattening that is not improving by six months of age

HEALING CORD

That little stubby bit of umbilical cord left over is kind of ugly, and many parents just don't want to mess with it. But there are no nerve endings in there, and you won't hurt the baby by touching the cord.

There is no single best way to take care of a newborn's umbilical cord stump. Many doctors encourage wiping down the stump with alcohol after every diaper change. This isn't necessary. Keeping the stump super-clean and free of normal skin bacteria will delay it from falling off. Clean the stump area if it gets dirty with stool, but otherwise the simplest and best approach is to leave it dry and leave it alone. With so-called "dry cord care," the stump will usually fall off within two weeks.

If you do notice some oozy wetness, or any odor from the stump, you or your pediatrician will need to clean the area. Lift the stump up gently and rub underneath the edge with a cotton swab moistened with alcohol.

! These red flags mean call your doctor:

- If the area around the stump looks red or swollen, or if it seems tender
- Oozing or an odor that remains even after a gentle clean with alcohol

HEALING PENIS

For boys who are circumcised, the penis can take several days to heal. During that time the end of the penis can look red and swollen, and a yellowish scab will appear. Just leave it alone and place gauze with petroleum jelly over the end of the penis to prevent sticking. If the circumcision was performed using a bell clamp, a ring of plastic will remain on the end of the penis for a week or so. Don't mess with it. It will fall off when the swelling goes down.

> ! These red flags mean call your doctor:
>
> - A penis that is becoming more red or more swollen, or that seems tender to the touch
> - Any persistent bleeding

HICCUPS

We don't understand why, but many babies begin hiccupping before they're born. These babies continue to hiccup for months afterwards. It doesn't bother the babies and no treatment is necessary.

IRREGULAR BREATHING

Newborns will sometimes breathe in a peculiar pattern. Respirations get deeper and quicker for a while, then seem to get slow and shallow, and then speed up again. For a few moments during the slow-and-shallow breaths, it may appear that there is no breathing at all. These babies are not struggling and otherwise don't seem to be in any trouble.

This pattern is called "periodic breathing," and is entirely normal in the first few months of life. You'll be more likely to spot your baby breathing like this just as he's falling asleep or waking up. It is of no concern, does not increase the risk of Sudden Infant Death Syndrome (SIDS), and is not something to worry about.

> ! These red flags mean call your doctor:
>
> - *Labored breathing.* Babies who are struggling to breathe will bob their heads, flare their nostrils, and allow their chests to cave in so that individual ribs are easily visible with every breath. They'll also breathe rapidly for long stretches of time.
> - *Blueness of the face, body, arms, or legs.* You may see blue hands or feet in a perfectly normal baby, but this blueness should not be on other parts of the body. Brief blueness right around the mouth, especially during a hard cry, is okay, but it should improve quickly when the baby calms down.

MOTTLED SKIN

Just as the surface vessels can clamp down and cause blue hands and feet, surface blood vessels all over the rest of your newborn can clamp down and cause a mottled appearance to the skin. You'll especially see this when a baby gets cold. If your baby appears mottled, bundle her up.

> ! These red flags mean call your doctor:
>
> - Mottled skin that is accompanied by fever, listlessness, or poor feeding

MURMURS

A heart murmur is an unexpected sound caused by turbulence in the flow of blood through the heart. In children and babies most murmurs are a normal part of the heart exam.

I wish we pediatricians had a different word to use for these extra heart sounds. Babies' hearts are very close to the front of their thin chest wall, making it easy for pediatricians to hear every little sound of blood flow. Besides, the flow is changing to accommodate the new life outside the mother and often there are extra noises as the flow pattern adapts. Overall, about half of all children will at some point have a murmur, and of course most of these kids have no heart problems. Still, when we tell the parents of a newborn that a murmur is present, it's hard to prevent the parents from becoming anxious. Sometimes, these murmurs are called "innocent murmurs" or "functional murmurs." I like to call them "normal."

If your newborn has a murmur, the pediatrician should explain what it means. If a murmur doesn't sound normal, further tests or a visit to a cardiologist is the next step. But most murmurs do not need any evaluation beyond your pediatrician's exam.

PEELING SKIN

Babies grow and develop entirely under water, and after birth that top layer of skin will flake off. You'll especially notice peeling at the wrists and ankles, where your baby is finally able to really stretch out the skin after birth. Much like a snake shedding its skin, the top layer is dead and no treatment is necessary as it peels off. It's safe to use a moisturizing cream, but it won't help peely newborn skin.

> ! These red flags mean call your doctor:
>
> - The skin underneath the peel doesn't look healthy and pink

RASHES

A newborn's skin can be a patchwork of rashes and spots. Most of these are entirely normal and will go away without any sort of treatment. Some of the most common newborn rashes are as follows:

- *Erythema Toxicum* (sometimes called Erythema Toxicum Neonatorum, or just Erythema Neonatorum) begins within a few days of birth and consists of blotchy red areas with irregular and ill-defined borders. Many of the spots will have a little white or yellow dot in the center.
- *Pustular Melanosis* begins as little pimple-like spots. They fade over a few days into small brown freckles.
- *Miliaria* can occur as red "heat bumps" or as tiny little clear dewdrops.
- *Milia*, or a similar rash called sebaceous hyperplasia, looks like little white dots on the face and nose.
- *Neonatal Acne* isn't present right at birth, but develops after several days. It looks just like teenage acne with red pimples, blackheads, and whiteheads.

Your newborn may have one or more of these rashes, and all of them can come and go for a while. None require any treatment at all. Other rashes, though, could indicate a serious problem.

> ! These kinds of rashes mean call your doctor:
>
> - *Petechiae* are little red dots under the skin that do not fade when the skin is stretched. A few of these can occur from pressure on the skin during birth; but petechiae scattered all over the body can be a sign of trouble and needs to be evaluated.
> - *Vesicles* are blisters on or under the skin. These can be a sign of significant infections. If you spot some, make sure your nurse or doctor sees them right away.
> - *Rashes* that appear when your child is acting ill—feverish, feeding poorly, or listless—need to be evaluated.

SLEEPING PATTERNS

Before babies are born, they're usually more active at night than during the day. Mom's activities—walking, talking, and moving around—seem to lull unborn babies to sleep during the day, and many prefer to be more active while mom is trying to sleep. This pattern naturally continues after babies are born.

To help your newborn start to figure out night from day in a way that gets parents some sleep, enforce rigid cues. During the day, keep things active and noisy. Talk or sing during feedings, and keep the lights on. Do the exact opposite at night—avoid talking or activity, and keep things dull and quiet. Also, try to follow a daytime pattern of sleeping, then eating, and then playing (rather than always feeding right before daytime naps). Soon enough, most babies will sleep more at night and use the daytime for more active play.

SPITTING

Babies, I think, are pretty smart. They know how to eat and breathe at the same time. They know how to get your attention if they need something, and they can recognize mom's face and voice within just a few days. But one thing they really don't seem to know is exactly how big their stomachs are.

Babies will often take too much from the breast or a bottle. Fortunately, there's a safe "backup"—an escape valve is built in to take care of the extra fluid when a baby overdoes it. Spitting up is a normal, safe way for babies to send part of the meal back up. Most spitting is of no concern. Just clean up, reassure your baby, and move on. Parents of frequent spitters should set aside money for a nice thorough carpet and furniture cleaning when their baby is finally past the spitting age.

Most babies don't complain when they spit up. These "happy spitters" don't need any treatment. If your baby does have periods of pain with spitting, it may be "gastroesophageal reflux disease," often abbreviated "GERD." More information about GERD and its treatment are in Chapter 19.

> ! These red flags mean call your doctor:
>
> - Spitting associated with pain, poor growth, trouble with breathing, or other worrisome symptoms.
> - Spitting that consistently flies across the room. An occasional big splash is okay, but if this is going on several times a day, your pediatrician ought to know.

SWOLLEN BREASTS

Both boy and girl babies may have some swelling of their breast tissue after birth from mom's hormones. Sometimes, a tiny amount of milk may even form. If your baby has swelling or some so-called "witch's milk," leave the breast tissue alone. Don't keep poking or squeezing the area.

> ! These red flags mean call your doctor:
>
> - Swollen breasts that are tender (painful to touch), warm, and red

TREMBLING

Lips, chins, arms, and legs all sometimes quiver and tremble in a newborn. This is of no concern. The easiest way to reassure yourself is to gently touch the trembling part. If the trembling stops while the limb is being touched, don't worry about it.

> ! These red flags mean call your doctor:
> - Trembling or shaking movements that don't stop with a gentle touch

VAGINAL DISCHARGE

Little newborn girls will have some sticky vaginal discharge. Sometimes, it can even appear bloody. This is entirely normal. Don't try to scrub it away or clean it up.

> ! These red flags mean call your doctor:
> - Vaginal discharge that appears pus-like or has an odor
> - Persistent bloody discharge

YELLOW SKIN (JAUNDICE)

Jaundice is a yellow color to the skin or eyes. It is caused by a chemical called "bilirubin" in the blood. To measure jaundice, a blood test can be used to determine the bilirubin level. Sometimes, a simpler test done on the skin can give a good-enough estimate.

Where does the bilirubin come from, and why do we worry about it? All babies are born with excessively rich blood. That is, their blood contains many extra red blood cells, to "soak up" oxygen from across the placenta. These extra red cells aren't needed after a baby is born, so they naturally break down. When they do this, the chemicals inside the cells are converted to bilirubin, which is cleaned out of the blood by the liver. But a newborn's liver isn't really very good yet at cleaning up the bilirubin, so it can build up in the blood and cause jaundice.

A little bit of jaundice won't hurt a baby; in fact, it may be a natural, good, protective mechanism. But if bilirubin levels get very high—especially in a baby who is already sick—it can damage a baby's brain.

Some things increase a baby's risk of having significant jaundice. Certain blood-type combinations between mom and baby can increase risk, as can premature birth, infections, or other health problems. We also see more jaundice in breast-fed babies, though the increased risk doesn't offset the overwhelming other advantages of nursing over bottle-feeding.

If your baby appears jaundiced or has risk factors, your pediatrician will probably arrange to have the bilirubin measured and monitored. To identify babies who become jaundiced after hospital discharge, the American Academy of Pediatrics recommends a follow-up visit a few days after discharge from the newborn nursery. If the level reaches a certain threshold, initial therapy is usually with blue fluorescent lights. Extra fluids from pumping or a formula supplement may be recommended. More severe jaundice will require more intensive therapy. If your baby's jaundice is recognized early and treated appropriately, there is very little risk of any lasting problems.

> ! These red flags mean call your doctor:
> - A worsening yellow color to your baby's skin or eyes
> - Poor feeding
> - Infrequent bowel movements in a baby less than two weeks old
> - Jaundice in a premature baby

Newborns are new. They're new to the parents, and they're new to the world. Many odd sorts of things can happen, yet most newborn babies are healthy and normal. The "newborn normals" in this chapter are meant as a general guide of what you can expect from your healthy, term baby. If your baby has special health circumstances including prematurity, you'll need to be extra wary. Even with a healthy baby, feel free to contact your pediatrician if you're worried about anything.

21

Healthy Eating for a Lifetime

You can find plenty of feeding advice for children. Grandparents and friends will be all too happy to pass along their own wisdom about how you were raised and how children ought to be fed. But your children will have their own ideas, too—and as you may have already discovered, a child will sometimes defy the most well-meaning plans. Expectations, pressure, and advice can make mealtimes a tremendous source of worry and gray hairs. I'm going to give you the simple, inside tips on how to virtually eliminate heartache and tension at mealtimes, and just about guarantee a nutritious diet for any child.

Newborn

Breastfeed, and do it frequently. The advantages of nursing are enormous both for baby and for mom. Unless there is a medical contraindication, and these are rare, just about every newborn should be breastfed exclusively. Some insider tips can help:

- During the first few days of life, newborns are not supposed to get much to eat. Parents, and even nursery nurses, often will say "that baby isn't getting enough." But mother's milk never comes in until a baby is two or three days old. If normal newborns needed plenty to eat from the moment of birth, then mom's milk would be right there, ready to go. It isn't. It's not supposed to be. The small amount of colostrum (often less than a few teaspoons per feeding) is all babies need at first.
- Some newborns are *impatient* for mom's milk. Avoid the word *hungry*, which is emotionally more powerful and worrying. For newborns who are impatient for their mother's milk to come in, a formula supplement given after nursing can help calm them down. But they don't *need* it.
- After your milk comes in, continue feeding frequently during the day. Babies need a lot of milk to grow, and what they don't get during the day they're going to expect at night. Frequent day feeds are the price you pay for longer stretches at night. It's worth it.

- As babies grow, they'll demand more milk. Mom's supply can increase, but will lag a few days behind. These "growth spurts" occur at unpredictable intervals. When babies spend a few days feeding more frequently, they're helping mom increase her supply. Growth spurts can be a rough and demanding few days, but once the milk supply increases your baby will resume her prior routine.

This section refers to normal term newborns. If you have a premature baby or are in a situation where the baby or mother has a health issue that may interfere with nursing, you'll need more specific guidance on how to keep your baby healthy as nursing is established.

Breast feeding is the ideal way to feed an infant, but bottle feeding is an alternative. When bottle-feeding:

- Don't bother with the more expensive bottle systems. They offer no important advantages, and many babies prefer the classic inexpensive bottles anyway!
- Follow the mixing and storage directions carefully.
- It is not necessary to boil or sterilize feeding equipment if you have ordinary city water service. Formula can usually be mixed using ordinary city tap water; ask your pediatrician if local fluoride concentrations are appropriate for a baby. Run bottles and nipples through a dishwasher.
- Most babies do great on milk-based formulas; soy formulas are also a reasonable choice. Avoid expensive formulas that claim to be better for fussy babies (see Chapter 19).
- Do not prop up a bottle to feed a baby while she's lying down. Hold her close, as you would while nursing.

INFANT (FOUR TO NINE MONTHS)

Start offering your baby foods like cereal, followed by veggies, fruits, and meat. When you start this process, it is entirely for fun and practice. For most babies, solids become an important source of calories by nine months. Offer an ever-widening array of choices, and avoid telling your baby things like "Oh, you don't like that." If your baby spits something out and makes a face, try it again in a few days without a reminder that it wasn't liked. Try to avoid showing with your face and body language that you don't like a food, either. Many "picky eaters" have a parent who never eats vegetables. Babies notice that.

Commercial baby food comes in little numbered jars. There is no appreciable difference between the consistency of "Stage 1" versus "Stage 2" jarred foods, so buy whichever size is more convenient and economical. Chunkier "Stage 3" foods can be started at anywhere from seven to nine months. Feel free to make some of your own purees of one or more table foods using a stick blender once your baby has tried the individual ingredients.

By six months children should have a sippy cup of water available with every solid meal (no juice, no soft drinks). Encourage your child to acquire a taste for water, and set a good example by drinking water yourself.

TRANSITION (NINE TO TWELVE MONTHS)

This is an important time, when babies change from mostly liquids to mostly solids as their energy source. Fortunately, this will happen automatically if you offer your baby good choices and stay out of the way.

As long as your baby is healthy and neither parent has food allergies, starting at nine months Junior can eat almost everything. The list of what a nine-month-old should not eat is short:

- No peanuts or tree nuts
- No raw honey
- Nothing hard that a baby can't squish between the gums

Other than these, you should introduce new "big-people food" every day. Good baby foods can be easily grabbed and should be cut smaller than the last part of your baby's thumb, past the knuckle. Some ideas:

- Canned beans
- Canned fruit or veggies
- Squishy meat, like meatballs or deli sliced turkey
- Bread or crackers
- Eggs
- Pasta
- Rice
- Any softish cheese
- Yogurt
- Any cereal—if it's hard, soften it in milk for a minute or so

Almost anything mom or dad is eating is fair game if it can be ripped into squishable bits. In fact, the best way to offer new items is right off of a parent's plate. Don't be afraid of salt, pepper, oregano, garlic, or any other "adult" flavors. This can be a fun time—enjoy sharing new food experiences with your baby!

During this transition to eating, encourage your baby to pick up her own food, feel it, and squish it around in her hands. It's messy, but important. Babies need to learn to anticipate what textures feel like, so they aren't so surprised or gaggy when trying new foods.

Try not to overreact to the occasional, inevitable gagging. Remember, gagging is not choking. The appropriate reaction to these two is not the same.

- Gagging is an involuntary expulsion of food from the upper esophagus and may be accompanied by vomiting. It does not have to scare the baby, and will not be a big deal as long as the parents don't overreact. Say something like "ooohh, that tastes weird! Take a sip of water to get it down."
- Choking is a frightening episode of breathlessness when food blocks the airway. If your child can make any sound at all while choking, it is best to offer only a little help with some gentle back pats. If your child is truly unable to breathe, strong blows to the back are the best first response to help clear the airway. Every parent should take a cardiopulmonary resuscitation (CPR) course to best learn what to do to help a choking child or adult.

Remember, nine to twelve months is a transitional period. Some babies will take to finger foods more quickly than others, but by twelve months most of your child's intake should be the same foods you eat.

TODDLERS AND PRESCHOOLERS

Feeding a toddler does not have to be an exercise in futility. There are three very simple rules. If you follow these, you and your child will be fine.

1. The parent's job is to offer appropriate foods.
2. The toddler's job is to decide how much of it he eats, or whether he eats it at all.
3. Normal, healthy toddlers will never starve to death, nor hurt themselves in any other way, because they don't like the food that is offered. (Unfortunately, children with developmental problems, mental retardation, autism, or other serious problems may not follow this rule. If your child is not neurologically typical, you may need more specific guidance for mealtimes.)

Mealtimes and snacktimes work the same way. Pick out a few items, ideally the same things that the adults are eating. Put them on a plate, or directly on a high chair tray. For some toddlers, it's best to offer food directly from your own plate. Put a few morsels in front of the child, then let him decide whether or not to eat them. Place a few more items on the tray when it is almost empty. If the child consistently refuses, say, the carrots, then don't put any more of those on the tray. Allow Junior to eat what he chooses from the tray for a reasonable amount of time—about fifteen or thirty minutes. At the end of that time, everyone gets up from the table, and mealtime is over. Any leftover food is cleaned up without any comments, and the child can be offered a wipe to clean himself up (with a little help). Don't offer any more food until the next planned meal or snack.

- Do offer appealing choices in small amounts.
- Do keep mealtime happy, and encourage your child to enjoy himself.
- Do encourage your child to feed himself, using his own hands or utensils—his choice.
- Don't force food.
- Don't coax, cajole, reward, or threaten.

- Don't repeatedly wipe up your child's mouth or clean up during the meal.
- Don't talk about what's left over afterwards.
- Don't offer more food until the next mealtime.

Your goal as a parent is to help guide your child toward good food choices throughout their lives. We know that children who are forced, coerced, or bribed to eat vegetables are less likely to choose to eat them when they are adults. You may need to sacrifice in the short term (that is, put up with a diet that contains no vegetables) in order to give your child the best chance of eventually learning to eat a varied diet.

The Insider's Guide to Feeding Myths

Kids need balanced meals. Medically speaking, nothing could be farther from the truth. It is true that kids need certain nutrients to thrive, but they certainly do not need a balance of different things at each individual meal. The belief that each meal should have a variety of food types is a relatively new idea, and really reflects an adult's sense of taste more than any biologic necessity. Don't fret if for some meals your child only eats three slices of cheese! All that matters is the long-term intake: what is being eaten over the course of weeks, or even months. A balanced *diet* does not require balanced *meals.*

Kids in developed countries are at risk for vitamin deficiencies. With a handful of specific exceptions detailed later in this chapter, vitamin deficiencies among normal children are not seen in the United States. Have you ever looked at the list of vitamin-fortified ingredients in any grain product or cereal? Even the pickiest children are awash in vitamins and minerals.

Kids need to eat their vegetables. An insider secret that needs to be shared: there is nothing crucial about vegetables. All of the vitamins they contain can easily be obtained from fruit or fortified cereals and grains. I'm not saying that you should not offer your child vegetables; I'm saying that it is not essential that anyone eat them. There is no reason to "trick" your child into eating vegetables, and it is even worse to bribe or force them to do it.

Vitamins are better from food than from a supplement. This just isn't true. The body could not care less if the vitamin C is from a nice juicy orange or from a chewable tablet in the shape of a bear. It's the same vitamin C! Of course, eating the whole orange does offer other benefits, such as other vitamins, fiber, and water. But vitamins themselves are identical whether from foods or supplements.

What about treats and sweets for a toddler? Occasionally offering these is fine if they are part of a meal that everyone is sharing. But too many children get their calories from soda, soft drinks, and sugary snacks. Save these for meals outside the home or special occasions. Don't include a "dessert" as part of every meal, unless by dessert you mean something healthy like fresh fruit.

Contingent feeding is a common way many families try to "get" their kids to eat something. A parent might say, "You can have your cookies if you eat your spinach first." In the short term, this might lead to more consumption of the foods parents want the kids to eat. But in the long run, contingent feeding is asking for bigger trouble:

- It psychologically increases the value of poor quality foods, while diminishing the value of healthy foods. Think about it. You only get cookies as a special sort of treat after eating something that must be terrible, right? Contingent feeding increases the future desire for the "bad" food, and decreases the future desire for the "good" food—exactly what you don't want to do.
- Studies have shown children who consume foods based on future rewards are much less likely to choose that food again in the future. "Okay, I'll eat this spinach—but never again, unless I get a brownie!"
- You end up fighting over the fine print. What exactly does it mean to take three bites? How big? How clean is a clean plate? Contingent feeding encourages children to argue and practice "gaming" the system.

Most toddlers do not like to eat the same amount at every meal. You'll be amazed at one breakfast—three bowls of cereal, plus applesauce!—but the next meal may consist only of licking the powder off of six goldfish crackers. It's the long-term view that's important. One meal may be huge, and loaded with protein; the next three meals may be "terrible." Toddlers will do just fine having one "decent" meal every other day! It can be frustrating to prepare meals for a toddler; it will only get worse if you let a child manipulate you into being their short-order cook. Stick to the simple plan: you offer, they decide. You'll both be happier.

> ☞ **The best way to know that your toddler is getting enough to eat is to review his growth chart regularly with your pediatrician. Children who track along a certain percentile that is similar to the way their parents grew are doing fine.**

You probably noticed that I didn't tell you how much food a baby or toddler should eat. Though you could find fairly exact numbers on the Internet, I suggest you not try to count calories, or keep track of individual nutrients. Follow these general guidelines, and follow your baby's growth. Normal growth means normal nutrition. Don't worry about the details or your child's exact day-to-day intake.

ROLE MODELS AND THE MEALTIME EXPERIENCE

The most important role models in the early years of your child's life are the parents. You need to show how good food choices are made. If you don't like milk, and your kids don't see you drink milk, don't be surprised if they won't touch it either. Likewise, if you have soda with every meal, what do you expect your kids will want to drink?

As your children grow older, other role models assume greater influence. What they'll see on TV is unrealistically thin models gobbling down sugary, unhealthy foods. Control what your kids watch by minimizing TV time and encouraging commercial-free videos over TV programming. This can have a lasting impact on your child's attitudes toward eating and food choices.

Mealtimes should be more than a time to eat. They're an important time for a family to be together and for children to learn social conventions. As often as possible, eat together as a family. Keep mealtimes pleasant and relaxed—don't use this time to review rules or berate a spouse. Turn off the TV, tell family stories, and talk about your day. Your children will learn how to share these family times together.

A Few Specific Foods and What They're For

A few specific food types inevitably cause concern and consternation when kids don't eat "enough" of them. What's in them, and why are we worried when our kids don't get them?

Vegetables are mostly water, and are very low in calories. They are a good source of vitamins, which can be found in many other places. They are also a good source of fiber, or what previous generations called "roughage." For those of you whose kids are less than regular with their bowel habits, increased vegetable and water consumption can help—but only if the child chooses to consume these things. Don't fight with a constipated child to increase vegetable consumption. It won't work, and you'll end up frustrated and upset with a child who is still constipated. For a better approach to constipation, see Chapter 12.

Milk is a great, cheap source of calcium, and is also fortified with vitamins A and D. Calcium and vitamin D are discussed below. Vitamin A is found in abundance in yellow or orange vegetables, as well as many fruits. For most kids, milk is the major source of calcium. If your child won't drink milk, you can use many other dairy or nondairy offerings to provide adequate calcium. Several good sources are listed later in this chapter. Children less than two should drink whole (full fat) milk; after age two any kind of milk is appropriate.

Meat is a good source of complete protein, which is seldom lacking in the ordinary diet of children in the developed world. It is also a good source of iron, though for many children fortified breakfast cereal has now surpassed meat as an iron source.

Three Micronutrients to Watch

In the developed world vitamin and mineral (collectively called "micronutrient") deficiencies are exceedingly rare. There are three exceptions:

Iron. Anemia from iron deficiency is common, especially in inner cities. Not only does dietary iron deficiency cause anemia, it also causes cognitive slowing and school difficulties. If your child's diet does not include red meat and fortified, iron-containing grains (usually cereals), you should either test for iron deficiency or give an iron supplement.

> ☞ **Liquid iron preparations can stain, so brush your child's teeth after administering them. One good-tasting brand of iron supplement is ICAR, which comes in liquid or chewable forms.**

Vitamin D. Rickets, a condition of poor bone mineralization, is usually caused by vitamin D deficiency. Children usually get adequate vitamin D from fortified dairy products, infant formulas, or sunlight exposure. Breastmilk alone is not an adequate source of vitamin D. Risk factors for deficiency include exclusive breast feeding, dark skin, and limited sunlight exposure. If your children are at risk for vitamin D deficiency, use a supplement.

Calcium. Children need a good source of daily calcium. For toddlers, milk alone is usually sufficient. (Sixteen ounces a day of whole milk will provide a day's supply of calcium, vitamin D, and protein for a two-year-old.) Calcium can be found in both dairy (cheese, yogurt), and nondairy sources (fortified juices and cereals, fortified soy milk). Some vegetables are rich in calcium, but it is less available for absorption than the calcium found in dairy and fortified products. If you're having a hard time ensuring adequate calcium, here are a few ideas:

- Add powdered dry skim milk to sauces, cereals, and baked goods. Powdered skim milk is nearly tasteless, cheap, and a great source of calcium. You can add it to almost any meal to bump up calcium intake.
- Try one of the chocolate-like calcium supplements, like Viactiv. This is a cube of yummy chocolate that happens to be loaded with calcium—more calcium than a glass of milk in each cube. Mmmmmmm, calcium!

Few children in the developed world suffer from an inadequate diet. Kids get their calories and vitamins. A more common issue than not getting enough food is that many children get too many calories, or too many foods that are sugary, processed, and unwholesome. Yet many parents become convinced that their children are not eating enough, and allow mealtime to become a frustrating experience of bribes, trickery, and hurt feelings. The most important goal in feeding a young child is to help imprint habits that will lead to a lifetime of healthy food choices. Set a good example, offer appropriate choices, and allow your children to make their own decisions about the amounts of each food item that they will eat. This is the best way to ensure a lifetime of healthy eating.

22

SIZE MATTERS: CHILDREN WHO ARE TOO BIG OR TOO SMALL

One of the most important issues pediatricians review at every checkup is a child's growth. Weight is a key reflection of a child's nutrition. Is he getting too much or too little of the right kind of food to eat? An unexpected fall in a child's height percentile—especially if it strays from the expected height based on parent size—can be an important indication of a serious health issue. Most important of all, head size reflects brain growth, and an unexpectedly small or (less likely) large head needs careful evaluation. Normal children do come in a variety of shapes and sizes. With a careful growth record, your pediatrician can make sure that your child is growing in a healthy way.

PERCENTILES: WHAT THEY MEAN

Your pediatrician should review your child's growth numbers at every checkup, including the "percentiles." This number is a rank, comparing a child to ninety-nine other children of the same gender born on the same day.

> Grace, at her one-year checkup, had a weight of 21 pounds (50th percentile, sometimes abbreviated 50% or 50%ile), length of 30 inches (75%), and head circumference of $17^1/_2$ inches (55%). That means if you lined up a hundred girls who were also one year old, she would be exactly in the middle of the pack for weight, at number 50. For her length at the 75th percentile, she would be longer than seventy-four and shorter than twenty-five. Her head circumference (55%) is very close to the middle as well. Her brother, who has always been slender, had a weight percentile of 10% at his one-year checkup. That means if you lined up a hundred one-year-old male babies in order of their weights, he's heavier than nine of them and lighter than ninety.

Weights, lengths, heights, and head circumferences are all plotted on graphs to determine these percentiles, comparing your child to other children of the same age and gender. Some doctors report percentiles as a range, say 50th to 75th percentile; others estimate a more exact number.

Most pediatricians use percentile charts generated from data collected from mostly suburban Caucasian babies in the early 1970s. They don't adequately reflect expected differences among ethnic groups, nor do they really show the kind of growth expected of nursing babies—most of those kids were bottle-fed. The charts are also not based on the size of a child's parents. Still, the graphs have stood the test of time and pediatricians feel comfortable interpreting them.

Most importantly, remember that the exact percentile number doesn't matter, unless your child is at the extremes of the charts. A single measurement anywhere from the 3rd to the 97th percentile is fine. It's the *trend* that's the most important. If your baby's head circumference goes from 80th percentile to 50th, then to 25th, then to 10th, there may be a serious problem that warrants an in-depth evaluation. But if your child's head circumference is 10th percentile, and always stays at about the 10th percentile, you've got nothing to worry about.

> ☞ **The most reassuring and dependable way to know that your child is growing correctly is to follow the percentile trend. A child who stays at about the same percentile from visit to visit is doing well.**

HEAD CIRCUMFERENCE

This measurement of head size is simple and reliable. It's a key way to know that your child's brain is healthy.

If your child's head is trending too big, the most common reason (by far) is that one or both parents have a big head, too. Though most pediatricians don't measure parents' heads, ask yours to check your own head size if your child's head is large. For men, the 98th percentile is 23 inches; for women, it's about the same, $22^3/_4$ inches. If a mom or dad (or both!) have head sizes at this level or larger, their child should have a big head, too. Parents can also look back at siblings' head sizes for reassurance. However, always be concerned if your child's head size is rapidly gaining percentiles, especially if there is any hint of developmental problems.

Heads that are small—that is, plotting below the growth charts at 0–2 percentile—are concerning. Even more concerning is a head that stops growing entirely. These kids may have a problem with brain development such as cerebral palsy. Your pediatrician should be aggressive in evaluating children with small heads and heads that are failing to grow.

LENGTH AND HEIGHT

Technically, length and height are not the same thing. When people stand, they're about a half-inch shorter than they would be lying down. To be consistent, length (lying down) is measured when children are less than three years old. Older than three, kids should stand for a height measurement.

Length in babies and toddlers is difficult to measure accurately because squirming children need to be stretched and held still to get an accurate number. More "aggressive" nurses can stretch out another inch or so! For the first couple of years, expect the height curve to be erratic and inaccurate. There should still be an overall upward trend, but the exact percentiles can vary from visit to visit and be misleading. By about eighteen months or so the measurements get more accurate and kids should be at a percentile that matches expectations.

How Tall Will My Child Be?

The midparental height is the best starting estimate. For boys, add the parents' heights in inches, plus 5, then divide that by 2. For girls, add the heights and subtract 5 before dividing by 2. Most children grow to be within a few inches of this midparental height as adults.

If a child's height is shorter than expected, or if the height percentiles are trending downwards, there may be a medical problem. Long-standing malnutrition will eventually affect height, though first you will see a more dramatic fall in weight percentiles. Some endocrine problems (for example, hypothyroidism), genetic issues (Turner or Down syndromes), chronic infections, and many other conditions can also contribute to poor height growth. Sometimes, it is a matter of "constitutional delay." This is another way of saying the child is a "late bloomer" who will catch up later. A careful history, physical exam, and sometimes blood tests and x-rays can confirm what's going on. Your doctor can refer your child to a specialist if a medical issue needs to be treated.

OVERWEIGHT AND UNDERWEIGHT

The weight (and to a lesser extent, the length) of newborns reflects the health of the placenta and mother during pregnancy. It doesn't predict how a child will grow during the first few years. In other words, big parents can have little babies, and little parents can have big babies. So the exact weight and length percentiles can trend up or down to some degree, especially in the first year of life, as babies "find" the correct percentiles that reflect how they're supposed to grow.

Still, a child who trends to the extremes of the chart (above 97th or below 3rd), or whose percentiles trend in an unexpected way, may be getting too little or too much nutrition. Review the principles in Chapter 21 to ensure that you're feeding your child in the most healthful way. An overly controlling feeding style is associated with an increased risk of both obesity and underweight. The best ways to prevent both of these conditions are to eat together as a family, follow commonsense advice about reasonable portions, and avoid overly processed foods. Overweight children should also have plenty of opportunities to burn off calories. The best way to encourage this is to turn off, or better yet get rid of, the television. Though families often insist on medical tests for overweight children, an ordinary history and physical exam will rule out the very rare medical conditions that lead to a child gaining too much weight.

For children who are thought to be underweight, the most common explanation is unrealistic expectations. In many cultures, chubby kids are thought of as more healthy and vigorous. Usually, when a child thought to be too skinny is measured and the weight curve plotted and followed, there is no problem at all. Remember a child who remains steadily at the 3rd percentile for weight is healthy and has no weight problem. Worry only about the children at the furthest end of underweight, and even then only if they're falling further and further away from the "normal" curve. For children who are genuinely underweight, the most common cause is an overly controlling feeding style. Sometimes, underweight kids are "sippers," who have developed the habit of suppressing hunger by constantly sipping on water or juice. Rarely, the issue isn't that the child is eating too little, but rather what happens to the food energy they're consuming. Some children have "malabsorption" from celiac disease or cystic fibrosis, for example. In conditions like these, the gut cannot absorb food energy—despite a big appetite, these kids don't grow well. Still other children may have an unexpected and hidden health condition that "burns off" a lot of calories. A chronic infection or heart disease can divert food energy away from growth. These issues are not common, but need to be investigated in a child who isn't gaining weight as expected.

An essential reflection of the health of any child is good growth. Though there is a wide range of "normal," the best way to make sure your child is growing well is to regularly visit your pediatrician for well health checks. The doctor needs to look at the overall trends of changes in height, weight, and head circumference to ensure that children are growing as they should.

23

COMMUNICATION REMEDIES

Parents are often frustrated that they just don't "know" when their child is sick. Sometimes they feel guilty if a child has been ill for a few days before an ear infection is diagnosed. At other times parents feel silly visiting the pediatrician for what turns out to be "nothing." By watching and listening, parents can learn how to tell if their children need urgent medical attention. Better yet, good communication skills can help many children feel better without a trip to the doctor.

TO KNOW IF SOMETHING IS REALLY WRONG: WATCH WHAT CHILDREN DO

By "really wrong" I mean something that needs the attention of a doctor right away. Approach this by paying more attention to how children act than to what they say. The bellyache expressed in the following conversation does not need to be seen quickly by a doctor:

> *Mom notices Gordon is acting blue, and didn't eat much supper.*
> *Mom*: "Gordon, is something wrong?"
> *Gordon*: "Yes. I have a tummy ache."

Clearly, something is bothering Gordon, but I wouldn't yet worry about a serious tummy problem. What mom noticed is that her son was acting blue, and she should follow up on that, not necessarily focusing on his tummy ache:

> *Mom*: "You do look down in the dumps. What's on your mind today?"

In the next situation, I would quickly rush to the emergency room (ER):

> Morris started complaining of his belly hurting earlier in the day. Now he is vomiting and doubled over in pain. Every time he takes a step, he winces; now he refuses to even get up.

That's a classic story for appendicitis, and Morris's behavior reveals how sick he is.

Another common situation might involve a suspected ear infection. As discussed in Chapter 5, ear infections usually begin during a common cold. If a few days into a cold a young child becomes more fussy or wakeful, you should suspect an ear infection and seek out a physician's evaluation in the morning. But if out of the blue, a child says "my ear hurts," I suggest you wait at least a day or two before having the ears examined. Be even more reluctant to worry about an earache that only appears after a parent asks about it. If it's bad enough to need medicine and medical attention, chances are the child will show it.

- *Most concerning:* When the child *shows* it. The child is crying, pulling at his ear, saying "my ear hurts!"
- *Less concerning:* When the child only says it. She's acting fine, but says "my ear hurts."
- *Not concerning at all:* When the child only answers it. For example, mom asks, "Does your ear hurt?" and the child responds "Yes."

Note that this advice applies best to developmentally normal infants and children, not to young babies. If you have any suspicion of illness in a baby, you should have the child evaluated quickly. Those little ones can fool you!

TO HELP THEM FEEL BETTER: LISTEN TO WHAT CHILDREN SAY

What? Didn't I just tell you to pay more attention to actions than words? *How children act* will tell you how sick they are, and whether they need urgent medical attention. But you have to listen to *what they say* in order to best help them feel better.

Let's continue the conversation with Gordon that started above:

Mom notices Gordon is acting blue, and didn't eat much supper.

Mom: "Gordon, is something wrong?"

Gordon: "Yes. I have a tummy ache."

Mom: "You do look down in the dumps. What's on your mind today?"

Notice mom doesn't focus right on the bellyache, but asks a good general open-ended question.

Gordon: "Everyone hates me at school."

Now we know why Gordon's tummy hurts. I'm not implying that Gordon is "faking" a tummy ache—to him, it really hurts. But sometimes a bellyache can have a very nonmedical cause.

Sometimes, you'll have to probe a bit deeper. The conversation could have turned out this way:

Mom: "You do look down in the dumps. What's on your mind today?"

Gordon: "I dunno. My belly hurts."

At this point, mom should give Gordon some time to discuss his pain.

Mom: "Where does it hurt? Tell me about it."

Mom should be facing Gordon, showing with body language that she wants to listen. Just listening and a gentle touch from mom or dad can help a child begin to feel better.

Gordon: "It hurts right here, like someone is pushing."

Mom: "When did it start?"

Gordon: "At school."

Mom: "What happened at school today?"

Gordon: "Everyone picked on me."

The conversation from there will focus on school, not on belly pain.

Even if the child doesn't directly discuss the stress, a parent can help a child feel better by suggesting a definite plan:

Mom: "What happened at school today?"

Gordon: "Nothing."

Mom: "Well, I'm sorry your belly hurts. Let's get you comfy on the couch, and I want you to hold this warm wet washcloth over your belly for ten minutes."

10 minutes pass.

Mom: "I'm glad you're starting to feel better."

Mom has said the magic phrase and gently removes the heating pad. The child goes off to play, having had some time to rest. He's feeling confident that mom knows how to help him feel better. That's a very powerful and therapeutic feeling.

Any body complaint can be caused by social stresses or psychology. Think especially about this sort of problem when a preschooler complains about any of the following symptoms:

- Bellyache
- Dizziness
- Headache
- Tiredness
- Sleep problems

There are more details about the various causes of these problems in other chapters, but it is important to not always assume any of these has a "medical" cause. More frequently, there are both biologic *and* psychological issues at work, and to help a child feel well, parents should be prepared to look for the stresses that are contributing to the symptoms.

A good scheme for listening and responding to a child's complaints follows these steps:

1. *Listen right away.* Don't force a child to get your attention with more dramatic or painful symptoms. When a child complains of a headache, it's best to quickly listen.

2. *Listen with attention.* Show with body language that you are listening and interested.

3. *Try an "explore question."* Often, a quick "How was school today?" type of question will get you to the root of the problem. If you don't ask, they won't tell.

4. *Encourage the child to discuss the symptoms.* Ask a few brief clarifying questions to allow the child to discuss the pain for a few moments. This allows the child to talk with your attention, which is therapeutic. This step should not last longer than thirty seconds or so. Use open-ended questions like:
    - Tell me about the pain.
    - Where does it hurt?
    - What does it feel like?
    - Why do you think it hurts?
    - What could I do to help it feel better?

   Avoid yes/no or leading questions:
    - Does it hurt right here?
    - Does your throat hurt too?

5. *Touch the child.* Touch is powerful and important. Try a kiss in the middle of the forehead for a child's headache. You'll be amazed how well it works.

6. *Attack the problem.* You need a firm, confident plan. It may include medicine (for example, a safe antacid for belly pain, or acetaminophen for a headache), comfort measures (hugging a heating pad), or resting in a certain way ("Lie here on your side for five minutes"). The plan should always include specific steps and be time-limited.

7. *Confirm the child is better.* Use a statement, not a question. Say "I am glad you're starting to feel better." This is a special phrase: it does not imply that the pain is all gone, it is reassuring, and it helps children feel better by making their parents happy. It's magic.

8. *End the encounter.* Gently change the subject and encourage your child to play, with a specific suggestion.
    - *Good:* "I'm glad you're starting to feel better. Go play with your sister."
    - *Better:* "I'm glad you're starting to feel better. Go play dress up with your sister."
    - *Best:* "I'm glad you're starting to feel better. Let me help you get your cowboy vest on to play dress up with your sister."

I'm sometimes asked, "What if it is really serious?" Families will not miss a serious illness by first following the scheme above. If the problem is something to worry about, children will show you with their behavior that they're truly ill. If after a few days symptoms persist in an otherwise well-appearing child, consider a trip to the doctor.

Reassuring factors (these are clues that pain is not caused by a serious medical problem):

- Pain in a vague location, or pain right in the belly button
- Symptoms that are difficult to describe or talk about
- Symptoms that only occur on school days, or are especially bothersome the few days after a school vacation

Concerning factors (clues that should raise your concern):

- Associated symptoms like fever, vomiting, diarrhea, or weight loss
- Symptoms that wake a child from sleep

Many symptoms have no definite medical cause, but are still stressful and upsetting to children. Watch how children act to help determine if immediate medical concern is justified, and listen to what they say to find ways to help alleviate the symptoms.

24

DISCIPLINE: TEACHING YOUR CHILD TO BEHAVE

A well-behaved child chooses to do the right thing. This doesn't occur automatically—young children are naturally petulant, noisy, and self-centered. We are born with ourselves in the center of the universe, an impression that is reinforced by parents who must cater constantly to their young babies. But babies become toddlers, and toddlers become children. Sometime during this transition, parents have to teach their children that they are part of a family. For a family to function and thrive there must be rules and expectations for everyone to follow.

I enjoy discussing behavior and discipline issues with families in my practice, and this chapter comes directly from what my patients and my own family have taught me. I've observed how parents handle their kids, listened to their frustrations, made my own suggestions, and followed through with many families to see what worked for them. Although the exact ways parents employ techniques of discipline vary, there are always five necessary components.

1. *Love*. Children must feel loved and secure. Without love, parents cannot teach their children anything.
2. *Clarity*. Children know the rules if they're applied clearly and consistently.
3. *Modeling*. Parents must not only demonstrate good behavior, but should show kids what to do when their own behavior isn't perfect.
4. *Rewards*. Friendly words and encouragement, along with occasional tangible rewards, are the best way to reinforce good behavior.
5. *Punishment*. Some parents ask about discipline *only* in terms of punishment, which is a mistake. Relying on punishments alone will not lead to long-term success. But parents should use effective punishments as one way to discourage bad behavior.

There are many good ways to apply these five components, and I encourage families to find their own solutions. Next time you're faced with a behavior dilemma with your own children, think about these five ways of approaching the problem. In the following sections I'll go through examples and more details about each of these five components, including practical ways of using them with your own children to prevent and treat behavior problems.

CHILDREN NEED LOVE

I know you love your children. But to little kids, a sense of love and security is fleeting. Changes in a family are one example of a time when love can become overlooked.

> About four weeks after baby Bradley was born, his three-year-old brother Hunter started having problems. He had been sleeping through the night; now he insisted on being rocked to bed. He started waking at 2:00 AM. At mealtimes, Hunter refused to eat what was offered and insisted on a different meal of his own. Drop-offs at the half-day preschool became a disaster of clinging, crying, and tantrums.

We know what triggered Hunter's difficulties: his new brother, and the realization that he's staying. His parents are exhausted and stretched thin.

I suggested that Hunter's parents approach this issue by first reinforcing their own time for love and affection for Hunter. Fortunately, this method really doesn't take any extra time. But for preschool children who are acting up when their family is undergoing changes, magic time can be fun, rewarding, and very effective.

One Method of Love: Magic Time

Magic time is a set period of time, usually fifteen minutes, where one parent must focus entirely on the child. It must begin with a special announcement—a parent looks at a clock and says, "Hey! It's time for magic time!" For the next fifteen minutes, that parent can do nothing but play with the child. Mom or dad should show with body language that they're really engaged—lean toward the child, and use touch to stay connected. No interruptions of magic time are allowed. After fifteen minutes, magic time has to end. An announcement has to be made with inflection and emotion: "Oooo magic time is over (*Say this sadly*). That was great! (*Happy!*) We'll do it again tomorrow! (*Even happier!*)" Magic time doesn't have to be with the same parent nor at the same time every day, but it has to occur every single day without fail. Extra magic time should never be given, even if the child has been extra good; magic time must never be taken away, even if the child has been terrible. Also, don't give magic time backwards—that is, you're not allowed to say "We've been playing for fifteen minutes.

That was your magic time." It doesn't count unless magic time is announced at the beginning.

Magic time is an expression of love. It's unconditional, it's fun, and it happens every day. For children like Hunter, 90 percent of their behavior issues can be solved with magic time alone. And you don't have to call it "Magic Time"—it could be "Paul's Time"—but it should have a special name to prove that it is special and magical.

If you have a particularly troublesome child, you may find yourself criticizing and correcting all day. This won't work in the long run. Your child has got to feel warm fuzzies at least most of the time in order for corrections to work. If children feel that they're always being criticized, there's really no reason for them to improve. You'll have better results when children feel warmth and love most of the time—that way when you do criticize, they'll quickly want to regain their warm fuzzies again. If they don't feel the love, they won't know what they're missing. If your child is spending a lot of time getting punished and getting dirty looks, reduce your expectations and concentrate your negative discipline strategies on the most troublesome behaviors. Once the top problems are solved you can then effectively apply your parenting skills to the smaller offenses.

CLARITY HELPS CHILDREN LISTEN

Being clear is an essential skill for parents. Your children should know exactly what is expected of them. They should know the rules, and they should know the punishment. They should know that your word is akin to the word of God: if a parent says it, that's the way it is. With clarity, your children will learn to listen.

Fostering this sense may not seem easy at first, especially if you've already developed some bad habits in communicating with your child. Keep two simple rules in mind to help establish clarity with your children:

Rule #1: Say what you mean.

- *Not effective:* "Natalie, why don't you go clean up your room."
- *Better:* "Natalie, please go clean up your room."
- *Best:* "Natalie, go to your room and put your toys in the box."

If you want your child to do something, tell them unambiguously exactly what you want them to do. Then, follow up and make sure it happens.

Rule #2: Mean what you say.

After you ask Natalie to go put her toys in the box, you need to make sure she does it. Don't repeat the request, don't threaten, and don't count to three. (Repeating, counting, and threatening tells the child you didn't mean it the first time.) If Natalie doesn't get up and start putting her toys away, silently but firmly take her hand and make her do it. If she does do it quickly as requested, then reward her with praise and thanks.

Children of different ages might not be able to handle the same sorts of commands. For an eighteen-month-old, it won't do you much good to say "Stop fidgeting in your chair." Kids of that age are supposed to fidget! You also couldn't expect a typical three-year-old to follow a complex instruction like "Put all of these toys away." In that case, breaking the command into several pieces, each one followed by immediate enforcement and praise, will be more effective *and* less frustrating for everyone.

If you can't enforce a command, don't make it. When you're starting the process of expecting your children to obey, help them succeed by not allowing any commands to slip by without enforcement. For instance, let's say you're carrying bags of groceries and there's a toy in your way. Don't ask your

> ☞ **Don't repeat yourself. Be clear the first time.**

child to move the toy for you—because if this request isn't immediately obeyed, you probably won't drop all of the groceries and make the child do it. Once your kids are used to listening to you, you'll see that unenforceable commands will start to work. But they've got to develop good listening and obeying habits first.

Using threats can diminish the clarity of your expectations, and will water down the effectiveness of any consequences.

- *Not effective*: "Stop jumping on the table, or we won't have dessert."
- *Better*: "Stop jumping on the table." Followed immediately, if child hasn't stopped, by a parent lifting the child off of the table. If the child persists in trying to jump, a punishment would be the next step.
- *Best*: The child already knows that jumping on the table isn't allowed, so the rule doesn't have to be repeated. A parent holds out a hand, the child stops, and the parent says "Thank you for stopping. I knew you'd remember you're not supposed to jump on the table."

If you do make a threat, be absolutely certain to follow up on it and enforce it. If you say "Stop that or there will be no dessert," then if the child persists for even an extra moment, dessert should be cancelled. Don't go overboard by making threats your child knows you won't enforce—"You do that one more time and we're never going to a restaurant again!" Who's going to believe that?

You may be giving your child too many instructions. If you're constantly asking your child to do things, he will tune you out. If you are having trouble with your child's listening skills, one way to practice success is to make fewer requests, but follow through to prove that you really mean the ones you do make.

Parents sometimes confuse details and explanations with clarity. Your preschool age child doesn't need complex explanations for what behavior is expected, and she doesn't need to be reminded of rules again and again. Once you've told her what the expectations are, stop talking about them and start enforcing them. Any statement to your child that starts with the phrase "How many times do I have to tell you. . . . " is unlikely to be helpful in changing a child's manners.

You may need to make sure your young child is listening *before* you give your instruction. Say, "Emma, listen to me, I need to tell you something." Stand in front of her, and make sure she meets your gaze before proceeding. A gentle touch on the chin before speaking can help a child focus on you. It's better to take these steps beforehand, helping your child to successfully listen.

The goal is to help your child learn to listen. At first, you'll have to exaggerate the clarity and precision of your instructions. Always follow through to make sure your instructions are obeyed quickly. Successful listening is a habit. Once your children get used to listening, your entire family will get along better.

PARENTS ARE MODELS

Many behaviors are learned by watching and copying. Almost all eighteen-month-olds know how to hold a phone—and most will even pace around and pretend to talk into it! Yet no parent ever explicitly sets out to teach their child how to use a phone. Children watch, copy, and do it. Good behaviors can be taught or reinforced the same way, just by modeling.

For example, family meals are a good opportunity to demonstrate good manners. Using utensils, drinking water, eating vegetables, and trying new foods are all desirable mealtime behaviors that your child is much more likely to do if parents set a good example that their kids can see. When children do not have an opportunity to eat with their family, table manners become much more difficult to teach.

Children have trouble handling frustration. They quickly forget to use words and can launch into a tantrum if they don't get their way. One way to help children learn how to handle these situations is to set a good example yourself. The message to your child isn't that you shouldn't get angry or frustrated, but that you should learn to handle these normal emotions in a good way. Your child should have a chance to see how you handle these situations: take a deep breath, count to ten, and settle down without losing your cool.

> ☞ **Both good and bad habits can be taught by example.**

Some kids get particularly upset if they make a mistake. They might cry if a teacher corrects them, or refuse to play a game if they aren't the best player. This is another good time to teach by example. Every parent should feel comfortable saying "Oops, I messed up" or "I'm not very good at this game, but I like to try." By saying these things and demonstrating that losing can be accepted gracefully, you can help your child become more mature.

Modeling alone will seldom fix entrenched bad behaviors, but it is an important tool for gently guiding your children toward better manners and more mature ways of dealing with stress. Together with a foundation of love and clear expectations, modeling provides a consistent message about what is expected. But to really fix a problem behavior, you'll need a more active approach. That's when teaming rewards and punishments will get you the results you need.

REWARDS ENCOURAGE GOOD BEHAVIOR

These final two elements are geared toward specific behaviors that you want to encourage or discourage. They work better as a team, though that isn't always practical. They also work better if used in a household that has already incorporated the first three elements of love, clarity, and modeling.

First, we'll discuss rewards. Also referred to as "positive reinforcement," a reward is something good given to the child after a desirable behavior has occurred. The "something good" that is used most often is praise—which can be very effective—or simply affectionate attention. Sometimes more tangible rewards like stickers or toys are appropriate. Food or candy rewards can work, but their routine use is not desirable as it leads to other unhealthful problems with weight and nutrition.

Bribes are different from rewards: they're given to the child *before* the desirable behavior. They are not as effective in changing behaviors as rewards, which are given *after* the good behavior. Ideally, you want your child to decide to do the right thing without a promise of a reward, and be sure to give extra praise when your child indeed does this. But when kids are younger you might need to let them see the carrot dangling:

- *Not effective*: "I'll give you a cookie now if you'll just be quiet while we're in the store."
- *Better*: "If you stay in the cart the whole time we're in the grocery, I'll get you a balloon afterwards."
- *Best*: "You were so good! I was very proud of how you stayed in your cart the whole time we were in the store. Here's a balloon!"

The most effective praise is specific, and given immediately after the good behavior:

- *Not effective*: "You were good at grandma's yesterday."
- *Better* (in the car on the way home): "I was proud of how good you were playing with grandma."
- *Best* (in the driveway heading away from grandma's): "That was great! I liked how you kissed grandma goodbye, and how you played cards with her. You made grandma very happy."

Some issues can be addressed with a more complex reward scheme:

Linnea is three and a half years old, and her mom would like to start encouraging her to keep her room cleaner. She set up a sticker chart on a calendar, so that every day right before dinner mom could do a room inspection. If fewer than three things are on the floor (including toys, clothes, shoes, etc.), Linnea earns a sticker. When she earns five stickers, Mom takes her to the dollar store!

This reward system lends itself to variations and tweaking as Linnea improves her room-keeping habits. For instance, mom could start to insist that fewer than three "floor things" would be needed to earn the sticker. Or, she could offer "double stickers" for days when Linnea did her cleaning up without any reminders. Later on, mom might require more stickers—say fifteen of them—for Linnea to earn a bigger reward, maybe a trip to the toy store to buy anything she chooses under $5. The goal is to start with small, frequent rewards that are gradually withdrawn as Linnea internalizes the expectation to get her room clean.

For Linnea, at age three, a reward system alone will be sufficient to encourage a cleaner room. But to really change behaviors in the strongest and most effective way, rewards for success can be paired with punishments for failing to improve.

PUNISHMENTS DISCOURAGE BAD BEHAVIOR

It is not correct to equate discipline with punishment. Discipline itself means "to teach," and it is a set of parenting skills including all of the methods reviewed in this chapter. But when many parents ask me "How do I discipline?" I know what they're really looking for is the most effective punishment to get their child to behave.

Punishment itself is only one part of a discipline strategy and it works best when combined with other methods. It should not be used for children less than a year old. Between the first and second birthdays, punishment should be reserved only to discourage physical aggression (see Chapter 25).

> ☞ **Rewards and punishments are most effective when used together.**

Learning how to appropriately punish your child can make discipline much more effective—and easier, too. The keys to using punishments are to be consistent, clear, and specific. Most of all, your children should learn that certain behaviors will *always* earn them a punishment. Always enforce the rules.

Punishments are best if they're immediate. For children older than three, they can be delayed somewhat if necessary, but the sooner the better:

- *Not effective*: "You're in big trouble when your father gets home."
- *Better*: "Once daddy gets home you're spending time in your room."
- *Best*: "To your room. Now."

The most effective punishments are natural consequences of the bad behavior:

- *Not effective*: "You broke your brother's toy. The next time he breaks one of yours, I won't replace it."
- *Better*: "You broke your brother's toy. You have to buy him another one from your allowance." (Preschoolers would not find this very compelling, but it might work for an older child.)
- *Best*: "You broke his toy. I'm giving him one of yours to keep now."
- *Also good*: "Because you threw the toy, it is going into time-out." (This last example would work even better if a little later you caught the child playing nicely and gave him his toy back, "I see you're playing nicely. I knew you could do that! Here is your toy back.")

Threats and warnings reduce the power of punishment, especially if you do not follow through.

- *Not effective*: "There will be trouble if you keep doing that."
- *Better, but still not very good*: "One more time, and you're going to your room."
- *Best*: "You hit your brother." (While simultaneously, and without saying anything else, taking the child to a quiet room for time alone.)

Some parents like to count off before punishments, which might help with a child who is overly impulsive and needs a little help keeping the rules in mind. But I've noticed that for most children all of this "One . . . two . . ." counting is really saying "You can ignore me for a few more seconds, but then I really mean it." Children's behavior will improve more if they know the rules are rigid and instantly enforced without a countdown.

Punishments should not be designed to "fit the crime," but rather to change the behavior. The kind of punishment will depend more on your own child than on what exactly was done wrong. For some children, a stern look will just wither them away with promises never to repeat the infraction, while other kids might need an hour of alone time to get the same effective result. You'll know your punishment is enough when you see that your child thinks twice before repeating the mistake.

Every punishment must be followed immediately by resuming a feeling of happiness and love. If your son feels like you're always angry or disappointed with him, it won't matter how he's punished.

- *Not effective*: "Your time-out is over. Why do you always do that? Never do that again!"
- *Better*: "Time-out's over. Come back in the room."
- *Best*: "Come here for a hug, time-out is over, I know you can do better next time." (Say this with genuine affection, no matter how naughty he's been.)

The single most effective punishment in most circumstances is removing the child from their happy play and away from their loving parents. For toddlers this is a "time-out"; for older kids, it's sending them to their room. I've heard many times that "Time-outs don't work," which is true if they're done incorrectly. Done well, time-outs are very effective even in the most stubborn kids.

A time-out should be immediate, with no warnings or threats. Say as few words as possible—ideally, none at all. In most cases, the child already knows the rule and knows it's been broken. For toddlers, take the child to the closest corner and hold them there, holding their head so they can't see you for about a minute. Alternatively, leave a toddler alone in their crib. For children older than two-and-a-half or three years, quickly take them to their room and leave them there on their own. Come back to rescue them when they've quieted down, or after five to fifteen minutes. Your first words after a time-out can be a brief retelling of the rule, said in a tone of support and love, "Now don't throw your toys, you can do better," along with a hug and a kiss. Every time-out has to be followed by a nice warm time-in, to really hammer home the point that the behavior earns them a very different sort of experience from what home is usually like. When 99 percent of the time is love and support, that 1 percent of cold-and-alone time-out is very effective.

What About Spanking?

A lot has been written about spanking, good and bad. Some people feel spanking in any form is child abuse; others feel there is a biblical injunction that encourages spanking.* To me, the main drawback to spanking is that it doesn't work very well. For most preschoolers, it might temporarily decrease the unwanted behavior, but parents who spank regularly find that it loses its effectiveness with time. Unlike other punishments, you cannot escalate spanking until it is effective again. Besides, when you consider that hitting and physical aggression are the main behaviors you want to stop in your child, parents do send a mixed message by continuing to model these behaviors when they spank.

If you do feel that spanking should be one of your parenting tools, there are important rules you should follow to keep your child safe. Don't spank when you're angry, don't hit with anything other than your hand, and don't leave a mark. Spanking will not be effective if used frequently. Spanking will not work at all under age two, as young children will not link getting hit as a consequence of their unwanted behavior.

Overall I discourage spanking because it is ineffective and difficult to do safely and correctly. More effective punishments and consequences should be used.

*The often quoted phrase is "Spare the rod, spoil the child," but the full verse from Proverbs 13:24 is "He who spares the rod hates his son, but he who loves him is careful to discipline him." Many scholars feel that this reference to "the rod" doesn't refer to a physical rod, but rather to firm and rigid rules. That is, the Bible may not be encouraging corporal punishment, but rather more consistent parenting.

Effective Discipline: A Summary

- Love, laughter, and affection are necessary. These should never be overlooked.
- Speak clearly and back up your words with immediate action.
- Don't waste words or rules on things you can't enforce.
- Don't talk so much about the rules, but rather enforce them all the time.
- Act the way you wish your child to act.
- Reward good behavior with specific praise, plus an occasional tangible surprise reward.
- Don't be afraid to punish. When a punishment is needed, do it without threats, warnings, or talking about the rules. Every punishment must be followed by a quick return of love and affection.

Discipline is a twenty-four-hour job that begins when your child is born. Using love, clarity, modeling, rewards, and punishments you'll be able to best teach your children how to behave.

25

FRUSTRATION, TANTRUMS, AND AGGRESSION

Ryan's parents were almost in tears as they described the transformation of their perfectly happy baby into a demon of a toddler. He used to be an easy baby, always playful, always smiling. Now everything is a nightmare—he screams when he doesn't get his way, and he seems unhappy most of the time. His parents just don't understand what led to this sudden transformation. They want their old Ryan back.

What happens to babies that makes children go from "I'm-just-happy-to-be-here" to "SCREEEEEECH" when they don't instantly get their way? And is there anything parents can do to get through this difficult period without pulling out their hair and swearing never to have another child?

WHY ARE TODDLERS SO FRUSTRATED?

Anger, frustration, and temper begin to develop in most babies between twelve and eighteen months of age. By that time, they're getting a clear idea of who they are, what they like, and what they don't like. What they haven't yet learned are the language skills to communicate well. They know they

☞ **Your toddler is more frustrated than you are.**

want the glass (the real glass, the one mommy uses—not that plastic thing with Winnie-the-Pooh on it), yet they can't seem to get that fact communicated instantly. When parents try to explain why a glass isn't such a good idea, it hardly helps a toddler settle down. Parents should continue to explain why things are the way they are, but cannot expect these explanations to work very well at this age. Phrases like "You can have a cookie—but after dinner!" are heard in every household, and are unlikely to make any toddler any more patient. The "terrible twos" begin at about eighteen months. For the next year or so expect frustration levels to be high and patience to be nonexistent.

Some toddlers are especially prone to problems with temper, frustration, and aggression. They may have a more rigid personality, or be anxious with change and unfamiliar events. Other children may be especially sensitive to touch, sounds, or their own body's sensations of hunger. Children who are less strong at communication skills—either late-talkers or children who do not yet understand their parent's speech well—are more prone to temper outbursts because of their frustration with not understanding or being understood.

WHAT CAN YOU DO ABOUT IT?

Two behaviors really stand out as the most troublesome manifestations of "twoness": temper tantrums and hitting. Before reviewing the best ways to handle these problems, there are some good general steps that parents of toddlers can take to cut down the overall frustration level.

Be aware of situations that bring out the worst in your child, and avoid them if possible. For example, many toddlers get especially ornery when they're hungry. Be prepared with little snacks, especially ones that include sources of slow-burning fat and protein calories rather than carbohydrates alone. Your child is also more apt to melt down on days when there wasn't a nap. Don't ask for trouble by going to the supermarket when you know your child is already cranky.

Foods and Moods

Some eating habits can certainly influence your child's mood. Even if your child doesn't ask for food or complain of hunger, you'll see more mood swings when children are running short of the fuel they need.

Different foods are metabolized more quickly than others. Sugary and starchy foods, including candy, juice, fruits, vegetables, crackers, and rice, are all digested quickly. These provide a quick energy boost. But the fuel quickly runs out, leaving the child even crankier than before! Foods that are rich in fat and protein are digested more slowly, so they provide a more slow-and-steady source of food energy. The best meals and snacks provide combinations of carbohydrates, fats, and proteins to deliver both quick and slow sources of food energy.

For instance, an apple alone won't keep energy levels up; smear it with peanut butter to make a better snack. A glass of juice is not a good snack, but if consumed along with some full-fat yogurt, your child will get a more substantial and long-lasting boost.

Practice success. You'll discover things that keep your child interested and cheerful, and you'll know which store you can run into for a few minutes to make her feel like you're running errands for her rather than for yourself. Good moods are infectious, and you'll want to help your child feel happy when you can. Children get used to being cheerful, and having positive experiences leads to more happy times.

Don't practice failure. If every time you go to the big department store your child has a meltdown, avoid going to that store for a little while. Children remember rough times, and after a few turns "practicing" their performance, they'll be more likely to repeat the show next time. Fortunately, memories are brief at this age, so a two-week break will usually allow you to reset your child's behavior.

Quickly and cheerfully honor requests that are "pretty good" and ignore requests that are rude. Ideally, we want all of our children to ask for things with a "please" and a smile. But don't insist on that, yet, during the frustrated toddler age. For now, anything short of screaming is probably a step in the right direction. If your toddler asks for something in a not-too-whiney way, go ahead and give it to him fast. Reinforce the lesson: if I ask for something nicely, I will get it. This goes for things you really might not want to give him—as long as it's reasonably safe, better to reward him for his fairly polite request than start up a tantrum. At the same time, ignore requests that are made with a yell, a whine, or a scream. As soon as your child learns you'll give in when she yells, you've lost the game. These lessons are tough for children to unlearn, so start early and be consistent.

Give your child choices. Babies don't mind if you decide everything—what they wear, which shoe to put on first, whether to sit in a high chair, which plate to use—none of these matter when a child is very young. Once a baby becomes a toddler, every one of these is a critical decision, and they want to be in control. So let them, within reason. When it's time to eat, hold up two plates and ask which one he wants to use. When it's time to get dressed, let her choose one of two or three shirts, and let her decide the order that the clothes will be put on. It's usually best to give children a limited number of choices. Hold up two shirts she can choose from rather than opening up the whole drawer for her to paw through. This isn't the time to micromanage outfits. Let children pick their clothes and let them enjoy the freedom of choosing other things, too. Of course, keep an eye on safety. No child can "choose" not to sit in their car seat! And sometimes you'll be in too much of a hurry to go through the choosing routine every time. But the more often parents allow children to make choices, the less they'll be frustrated at the times when they don't get to choose.

TEMPER TANTRUMS

All toddlers will have occasional temper tantrums. You can't stop all of them, but you can discourage them from happening in the future. With some patience and a good action plan, most children will stop having temper tantrums by age five.

Temper tantrums can be broken up into four stages, and how you handle each stage is different:

1. *Between tantrums.* Life is calm here. But try to avoid situations that are likely to bring out a tantrum. A tantrum avoided is a good thing.
2. *The pre-tantrum.* The tension is building, and you can see one coming. The best thing to do here is distraction. Don't give in to what your child wants (that will encourage future tantrums), but if you can distract her with something else, or just break the tension with some tickles, you've done well. Unfortunately, the "pre-tantrum" may last only a few seconds, and you may not have time to recognize a pre-tantrum and intervene before the next stage.
3. *The tantrum.* The yelling, the lying on the floor, the hysteria: as far as your child is acting, it's the end of the world, and it's your fault. Have no guilt and no anger. Just let it go. Don't try to help, don't soothe, don't punish, and don't try to teach. Take a few deep breaths yourself, and let it burn out. As long as your child is safe, you can even just walk away.
4. *The post-tantrum.* This includes a whimpering cry, wet and pink puffy eyes, and irregular gaspy inhalations that make it difficult to talk. Pick up your child, hold her close, and whisper, "I'm glad you feel better. I know you don't like to lose control. I'm glad that's all over." Say these things to help your child feel better, and also to remind yourself that a temper tantrum isn't deliberate. Your child probably feels worse than you right now.

To review: Between tantrums, avoid. Pre-tantrum, distract. During tantrum, ignore. Post-tantrum, reassure. Tantrums are a manifestation of a loss of control and frustration that your child doesn't have the maturity to deal with—yet. With patience and a consistent reaction to tantrums, they'll get fewer and farther between as your child grows.

 You can't teach a toddler anything in the middle of a tantrum.

AGGRESSIVE BEHAVIOR

Many frustrated children will hit, pinch, kick, or bite when they're really mad. Parents typically start to see these behaviors from fifteen to eighteen months of age. Like tantrums, aggression is another manifestation of a developing sense of frustration and temper. For many families, this is the first real discipline challenge. It is the first time punishment should be used as part of a strategy to teach your child to behave.

Kids do not inherently want to be aggressive, and don't like feeling frustrated and out of control. However, aggressive behavior can quickly develop into a habit. They can quickly learn that their behavior will get them what they want, or at least get them attention (this is of course being what toddlers really want most). Fortunately, a consistent approach will usually stop aggressive behavior in about two weeks. You need to make sure that all caregivers know the plan and everyone will enforce these rules equally and consistently.

Make sure you aren't modeling aggressive behaviors, even in fun. If you're trying to stop your child from biting when mad, you need to stop any sort of "nibbling" fun. Likewise, sometimes parents like to play "little boxer" with a toddler, but that sends a mixed message if you're trying to create a "no-hit" household. Spanking or "popping" your child's hand will not help stop a child from hitting, and may lead to an escalation of the behavior. You certainly don't want an "arms race" where you and your child have to hit each other harder and harder to make your point. Also, review the background ideas in Chapter 24 and the beginning of this chapter for general information about decreasing the tension and frustration in your household as you begin the process of teaching your child not to be physically aggressive.

Eliminating aggressive behaviors requires a quick, consistent response. In this example, I'll refer to hitting, but this response plan should be used for any aggressive action (biting, kicking, pinching, or slapping). Don't try this method to extinguish dirty looks, or "almost hits." The method works best at stopping actual physical actions.

1. Don't do anything until and unless your child hits. That is, don't try to warn him before he hits that he shouldn't do it. He already knows, and repeating rules is never a good idea.
2. As soon as your child hits, immediately hold him up in the air with your hands under his armpits, facing you. Say exactly two words: "No hitting." Say these words with anger and your "mean face," but remain in control. Don't yell it.
3. Within another second, turn him around so he is not facing you. If your child is older than two, you may need to march to the nearest corner and hold him there. If he's too big to hold up in the air, sit down and give a hug from behind. This is not meant to be a loving and supportive gesture; this is meant to demonstrate that you can—and will—physically control him if you need to. Hold him in this "mini time-out" for twenty seconds for a toddler, a minute or two for a two-year-old.
4. Turn him around, and let him see that all of the love is back on your face. You cannot remain angry at this point (that dilutes the message). Repeat your instruction, "no hitting," but this time say it in a sweet and loving voice.
5. Put him down. It's over. Do not remain mad and do not show with body language or in any other way that you're still disappointed or upset.

You and every other caretaker must repeat these steps, exactly, every time Junior takes a bite or hits. Do not escalate the punishment, and do not warn when one is coming—just do it, every time. In fact, if your hands are full or if in some other way you can't follow the "hitting" plan, it's best to ignore your child's hit. Never use an ineffective warning or halfway punishment. That will reinforce in his mind that you are not in control.

Temper tantrums and hitting are two manifestations of the frustration that many toddlers and young children feel. They often can't communicate very well at this age, and are not very good at accepting rational explanations. The frustration itself is normal and is a part of growing up—there is no way to completely eliminate frustration from your child's life, or from your own. You should help your child learn to deal with frustration with love and compassion. However, you should not tolerate the antisocial behaviors that occur when children are frustrated. Action plans to decrease both temper tantrums and hitting will mold your child into a better person, and in time will decrease the frustration level for everyone in your home.

26

POTTY TRAINING

Most children are happy to learn to use a potty when the time is right. Often, minimal work is required by parents. Some general support, a few high-fives, and a willingness to clean up a few messes will get the job done. For some families, though, potty training turns into a struggle. Children can become constipated and miserable, and parents may be at their wits' end. None of this is necessary, and all of this can be prevented by keeping a few simple truths in mind.

> *Truth #1: All children will learn to use the potty.* Neurologically normal children do not go to kindergarten in diapers. Sometimes parents need to take a break from all potty efforts. Eventually, the training will get done, often without further parental coaching.
>
> *Truth #2: Parents cannot make children use a potty.* Kids have control of their anus as well as their bladder. You cannot make a child defecate when you want them to or where you want them to. Children can—and will—make themselves sick if you try to force this issue.
>
> *Truth #3: It doesn't matter how old children are when they learn to use the potty.* I know there is at least one prominent national columnist who thinks parents are failures if they don't get their children trained by a certain age. This is a misguided bias that puts unnecessary pressure on parents and kids. Using the potty is one skill—one of many hundreds or thousands of skills that children learn. It is not fundamentally more important than learning to tie shoelaces, use a computer mouse, or eat with a fork. That the exact age of training in this one skill is so crucial to some parents, schools, or columnists is silly. That's not to say that a child's age isn't important in some ways. In the next section, I'll go through potty training tips based on what works best for different aged children. A child's age affects the style of teaching that is most likely to succeed. But in the end (ha ha!), it's going to happen. It doesn't matter exactly when.

POTTY TRAINING BARRIERS

Parents do have an important role to play in potty training. A few things may prevent or delay potty success at any age, and parents need to be aware of these things to avoid problems.

- Constipated children will not potty train. If stools are hard and painful, children will try to hold them in. Stools held back will get bigger, harder, and more painful. This can lead to an intensifying spiral of constipation, holding, pain, and more constipation. If your child has painful stools, review Chapter 12 and work with your pediatrician for treatment until the painful memory is gone. Do not resume any efforts to train until constipation is over and forgotten.
- New stressors can stand in the way of any developmental step. Don't try to potty train when a new sibling has just been born, or just when a child is first starting preschool. That's asking for trouble.
- Unrealistic expectations may be felt from a parent or another caregiver. Children need to feel that they're successful, even if they can only perform some of the steps of using the potty. A spouse might not feel his son is getting much done if he "just sits there," but being able to sit still and wash hands afterwards are two important parts of the whole potty experience, and should be praised and supported. Comments like "that doesn't count, you didn't do anything!" are not helpful.
- Too much overall negative discipline will not make a child eager to please. If you've fallen into the habit of using too many time-outs and restrictions of privileges, rather than positive reinforcement, you will not have a pleasant potty training experience. Review Chapter 24 for more about using a balance of positive and negative discipline tools to help teach your child to behave.
- Avoid negative vibes about potty and stool issues. Parents who refer to what's in the diaper as "stinky" are more likely to have a child who runs and hides to have a bowel movement, rather than a child who is eager to tell mommy before it happens. Avoid negative faces or words when discussing stool, urine, or other potty things.
- Punishments have no role whatsoever in training children to use a potty.

SUCCESSFUL STRATEGIES

Some important pointers and strategies will help any family get through potty training.

It's got to be fun. Some authorities write about potty training as such a grave and important issue! Let your little boy pee on a tree outside. Let a child sit on a potty chair in the living room. Buy colorful underwear, and let children play with them on their heads if it

☞ **Fun helps.**

makes the occasion more special. Sometimes, letting children know about the secret "poopy party" out in the sewer—the magical place where mommy and daddy's poopies go to play—can provide a gentle push to encourage success. Not all children will fall for this, of course, but keeping it light and fun is more likely to be successful than acting like a pooping drill sergeant.

Practice success. There are many steps to a successful potty trip:

1. The child has to know they've got to go
2. The stool or urine has to be held, at least for a few moments
3. Clothes come off
4. Diaper comes off
5. Sit (Boys can stand, but it's simpler and less messy if they sit!)
6. Relax and push (This may sound easy, but it's not: how to simultaneously push down with the abdominal muscles while relaxing one's anus and pelvic floor is a skill that children do not know automatically.)
7. Wipe
8. Get clothes back on
9. Flush
10. Wash hands

That's a lot of steps, when you think about it. Your child is moving toward complete potty training when he or she can do *any* of these steps. Every time one or more of these steps are practiced successfully, your child is nearer to getting them all learned correctly. It is far better to "practice success"—that is, praise and reward practicing any of these—than to criticize or push for more steps to be done. A toddler should earn at least praise for a quick squat-n-flush, even if no actual "output" occurs. It's a step in the right direction.

Don't go overboard with the rewards. It's one thing to offer a sticker or a small candy treat, but a trip to Disney World for a poop is overdoing it. Don't make children think that potty training is the most important thing in the world by making the reward extravagant. Nice little special rewards are more

> ☞ **Frequent, small, surprise rewards work better than big planned rewards.**

effective than huge ones. One of the best rewards I know of is to get a number of tiny little items—cheap plastic dinosaurs, a few pieces of candy, that kind of thing—and gift wrap each one in a little package. A child, after completing a successful trip, can get to pick one of these out of a "grab bag." Unwrapping a small reward makes it more special!

AT ONE YEAR: LET CHILDREN IMITATE

Have you noticed that most two-year-olds know how to wash dishes? They'll hold the dish in the sink, wipe it with a sponge, and spend thirty minutes wasting a whole bottle of detergent! No one taught them to do it; they just like to copy the behaviors they've seen parents do. When children reach their first birthday, it's time to start potty training by allowing children an opportunity to copy their parents and older siblings.

Starting at about a year, or whenever children start walking, leave the door open when you go to the bathroom. Let toddlers wander in and see what's going on in there. After they've watched the routine for a few weeks—they're usually very interested—put a potty chair next to the toilet for them to sit on. Don't pick them up and put them there, but instead just wait and they'll usually imitate you when they see you sitting. (Dads may need to spend a few months sitting, too. You probably don't want your little toddler boy standing to practice, at least at first. That's what the backyard is for!) Once a toddler gets used to sitting when you do, calmly take off their pants and diapers after you pull down your own pants and underwear. Again, don't make a big deal about this. Let them copy and practice rather than doing steps for them.

Sometimes, toddlers will imitate every one of the ten steps listed above. You may have a potty trained eighteen-month-old without having done much of anything! More often, children of this age will imitate only some of the ten steps, leaving out some crucial parts. No matter. Any steps that are learned through imitation are steps in the right direction, and they'll leave you and your child closer to the finish.

AT TWO YEARS: PRACTICE AND REWARD

By age two, you may need to take a somewhat more active role in training. Don't pester your child, but set aside at least one time a day to encourage a potty trip. To increase your chance of success, pick a time about when a bowel movement often occurs. Be positive and reward any correct steps with praise. Sometimes, a "tiered" reward system helps—the child gets one M&M for any attempt, two M&Ms for peeing in the potty, and three for pooping! (Keep the M&M bag in view, and use these rewards to also teach the names of colors.) You might try the "grab bag" rewards listed above; if Junior indicates he has to go, and makes it to the toilet in time, he gets a grab bag item! Be sure to choose a "reward threshold" that your child can easily reach, at least most of the time. Move that threshold up to a slightly tougher level once your child has mastered early steps.

If your child starts to resist training efforts, it is better to put them on hold than to fight. You can even say something like, "I can see you aren't ready yet to use the potty. That's okay. Let's color instead!" Don't focus on the "step backwards," but find something else to do. Within a few weeks, most children will be willing to go back to practicing as long as they aren't pressured.

Although it's not necessary, some families like the guidance of working along a particular timetable to reach individual goals. This can be a nice, gentle approach for children who are not particularly outgoing or interested in forging ahead on their own. Although exactly how you break up the steps won't matter, the idea is to start with something your child is already doing, adding a new step or expectation about once a week. If the child balks at any step, you have to back down. As an example, here's one way a family broke training into weekly steps:

Week 1: Starting with the skills he already knew, Sam gets praise and affection for sitting on the pot with his clothes on and washing his hands afterwards. Sam had already learned to do these things by imitation. If your child doesn't want to sit on the pot just yet, that's fine. For a preliminary few weeks, let him sit on the potty in silly situations—in the living room, or during a snack.

Week 2: Mom noticed that Sam really was only sitting for a few seconds. So this week, she encourages him to sit a little longer by reading a story.

Week 3: When mom goes to the bathroom herself, she asks Sam if he wants to take his pants off, too! He's reluctant at first, but by the end of the week he starts pulling them down himself.

Week 4: Sam is happy to sit on the pot, but doesn't seem to connect sitting with any further production on his part. This is common. To help Sam connect the dots, mom shows him where poop goes. After Sam has a poop in his diaper, mom takes him to the bathroom and drops the stool into the toilet, explaining, "This is where the poopy wants to go!" If Sam wants, he can flush the poop down and earn more praise.

Week 5: He's happy to follow the steps, but yet to have a bowel movement on the potty. Mom has Sam start spending just a little while each day with no pants or diaper. During this time, they play in a room with no carpeting, and move the potty into the same room to serve as a little reminder. There are accidents, and at first Sam is scared and upset when he soils himself. Mom takes a break for a few days, but then Sam asks for some special potty time. It works! Mom, who has been praising Sam for all of his false starts and tries, gives him just a little extra praise, and shows him the new "grab bag" of little wrapped goodies. She tells him he can have potty time every day for as long as he likes, and every time he puts his pee or poops in the potty, he gets a new grab bag goodie! After a few successful days, they take a trip to the store to pick out some cool underwear. There are a few more accidents, but Sam can now spend all day out of his diapers.

Successfully potty training a two-year-old child requires persistence, gentle encouragement, and a little luck. Some kids just won't be ready or willing to train at this time. This isn't a bad reflection on the child or the parent. But as your child reaches his third birthday, the emphasis on training should change from practice to patience.

AT THREE YEARS: SET THE STAGE AND WAIT

Just about all three-year-olds know how to use the potty. They know how to hold their stool or urine, and they know where it is supposed to go. If they care to try, they will get it right. But many of them just aren't ready (or willing) to take the plunge and do it.

You already know you can't make them do it, and you've probably realized a three-year-old doesn't need to practice the individual components anymore. Any reminders, nagging, or cajoling will only delay the process. All children will come to the realization that it's nicer to use a potty than soil their diaper, but if they're caught in a power struggle with their parents it will take longer. The best method for potty training a child from about three years of age and up is different from the way you approach a typical younger child. There's no week-to-week plan, just some ground rules to encourage success:

- Look over the section above on barriers and problems. Be certain your child isn't constipated, and that there are no external pressures, negative vibes, or punishments surrounding potty issues.
- Have a nice chat. Make sure to tell your child that you know she can do it, but that you also see that she isn't ready yet. Tell her you're okay with that, and you're proud of her, and you know that once she's ready she'll be great at using the potty. Tell her you won't be giving her any reminders to use the potty anymore, and you're going to stop all discussion of potty issues. Pretend you don't care about these things anymore, because you know that she already knows what she needs to know. You should only have this talk with your child once.
- Make sure that you and all caretakers follow through on what you've told the child. No reminders, no potty talk, no practice runs. Don't even go into the bathroom to "help" unless the child asks you.
- Make it easy for the child to get to and use the potty. You might leave it in a central room rather than in the bathroom, or set up some small steps so your child can climb onto a ring on the full-sized toilet. If you want your child to use a toilet rather than a potty seat, you should also provide a step for your child's feet so they don't dangle.
- Set up a simple, easy-to-remember incentive program. You can even ask your children what they think would be a nice reward for using the potty, and offer that if it's reasonable. Later, I'll review the best rewards to motivate children.

UNWILLING TO WAIT? AN ALTERNATIVE WAY TO APPROACH A LATE TRAINER

Every child will train eventually if the simple rules above are followed. After a point, no further "practice" is needed. Children get so used to all of the attention for *not* performing that they don't see any reason to get it right! By ignoring nonperformance and stopping all reminders, children will eventually come around to using the potty and earning more affection and rewards that way. Besides, no child actually likes to walk around in soiled diapers or underwear.

But if you're unwilling, or just unable, to completely ignore your child's lack of progress in the potty arena, you're going to need a backup plan. If there is any hint of pressure or "just checking," your child will continue to delay training. For these families, a more involved approach is a better way to go. This approach is in a way similar to how you would ordinarily train a young child, but the individual steps are even smaller and more technical for a child older than three.

Start with where you are, or where the child is willing to be. Reward that, and only when the step is mastered do you change the expectations ever-so-slightly to get a single baby step closer to success. You don't necessarily have to take a step each week. In fact, each step can be longer or shorter, but should always last until the child is 100 percent comfortable with the current step. Be sure you've already told the child that you know he's not ready to do it all just yet, you're proud of the steps he does do well, and you know he'll be able to do everything just right when he's ready.

> *Week 1*: Jacob is now having a bowel movement while he hides behind the couch. This tells his parents he knows when it's going to happen, and can hold it long enough to get back there. His parents offer him a deal: if he comes and tells them afterwards that he's had a poopy, he gets a reward.
>
> *Week 2*: Jacob's parents praise him for telling them afterwards. But there's a new rule: "If you can just shout out while you're having that poopy, you get a new reward!" They really can't expect him to do more for the same reward, so parents have to be a little creative this week and every subsequent week to come up with something new.
>
> *Week 3*: Now Jacob has to tell his parents in advance, or at least while walking behind the couch.
>
> *Week 4*: Jacob's parents move the couch to near the bathroom. Jacob doesn't really have to do anything differently.
>
> *Week 5 and beyond*: Each week gets a little closer. First, Jacob has to stand behind the couch right near the bathroom door. Then, he has to stand just outside the bathroom door. Then, he has to touch the bathroom door; next, he has to stand inside the bathroom (but still not near the toilet). The next few weeks he'll have to stand ever-closer to the toilet, until a week is spent touching the toilet, then finally sitting on the toilet in diapers, and then even pooping through a slit cut into the diaper. Finally, he's expected to actually poop into the toilet!

This whole time, Jacob gets praise and rewards for what he does do right: washing his hands, or holding it in while he goes behind the couch, or any of the other steps short of actually pooping into the toilet. It's difficult to keep up the praise week after week, but it does work. Many times, children will just jump to the finish line once they're tired of the baby steps. But if you're going to train a child with baby steps, it may take a while. Be prepared for a long journey!

SETBACKS

Your child has been successfully trained, and starts to have accidents again. Review the barriers listed above—is she constipated? Is there another medical problem like a urinary tract infection or diarrhea? Could she be frightened about a family change?

If there isn't a medical problem and the family avoids punishments and ugly looks, occasional setbacks will be brief. You may need to reintroduce some incentives, or go back to an earlier step of success and rebuild from there. One thing I would be reluctant to do is allow a child who had been successfully trained to resume wearing diapers. Just leave the underwear on, and help the child clean up after accidents without any punishment. If it's an older child with only urine accidents, expect the child to clean up after herself and change her own clothes—and earn a reward for doing that. However, if your child is holding her stool in, you may need to offer to put her back in diapers, at least for as long as it takes her to relax and have the bowel movement.

INCENTIVES AND REWARDS

Incentives and rewards are very useful for reinforcing behavior that you want to encourage. You'll need to think about your own child's habits and preferences, but some general rules about rewards will help guide you to the best choices.

- Rewards are effective, but bribes are not. Rewards are given *after* the good thing is done, and rewards will increase the likelihood that more of the good things will happen in the future. A bribe is given before the behavior— like saying before going into the store, "Here's a candy bar, now behave yourself." Bribes do not work as well as rewards. It's far better to hold onto that candy bar until later, after a successful trip.
- Rewards aren't necessarily needed every single time, and in fact repetitious or expected rewards will lose their appeal. Mix it up and give unexpected rewards.
- A good way to give a "big" reward is to give time with a favorite new toy. Once you give your child a video game for a successful potty trip, it can no longer be used as a future reward. But if you say, "You get a half hour of play time on the video game!" you'll get more mileage. Offer rewards of more time in the future.
- Food rewards are a mixed blessing. Some families don't like to mix eating and bathroom behaviors, and it isn't really a good idea to overemphasize candy and junk food. I prefer to make food treats more social—like earning stickers that count toward a trip for ice cream with dad. But sometimes a few M&Ms can get you pretty far!
- *Extra* special time with mom or dad can be a great reward, but don't withhold these activities as a punishment.

NIGHT TRAINING

About half of four-year-olds are dry through the night, and from that point forward about 15 percent of children will begin to stay consistently dry each year. Children who night-train later are usually the deepest sleepers, and often have one or both parents who were late to stop wetting the bed when they were children.

Staying dry through the night has nothing to do with learning, training, discipline, or how hard children are trying. It will occur, automatically, once the nervous system develops to the point where kids can sleep soundly while still paying attention to feelings from their bladder. The soundest sleepers just don't wake up, no matter how full their bladder becomes.

There is no need to "train" a child to sleep dry through the night. You can leave your child in pull-ups, or change the sheets every morning. By age three or four, a child should be able to help with the morning routine, either by stripping the bed or by putting the wet pull-up in the trash. Be very matter-of-fact about this routine, and do not give children the impression that it's their fault they're wet, or that you're anxious for them to learn to be dry.

Potty training is one of many important skills that your child will master. Teaching begins by setting an example, and later by practicing success. As children get older, it becomes more important that you stop reminding and cajoling them to use the potty—they'll get it eventually, and parental pressure will only delay success. Though the timing of training isn't crucial, parents can take an active role to encourage success starting at an early age.

27

SIBLING QUESTIONS AND ANSWERS

WHAT'S THE IDEAL AGE DIFFERENCE BETWEEN SIBLINGS?

Think about your own family and your own expectations. You may have had a particularly warm relationship with a sister who was close to you in age, or you might remember fighting with a sibling who was very much younger. These memories inevitably color how we think of our own children, but that isn't necessarily wise. Children sometimes fight, and children sometimes get along—but it isn't always because of birth order and spacing. Their own personalities, skills, and developmental status may have more influence on their relationships than the differences in their ages.

Consider not only the relationships between the children, but also your relationships with your children, spouse, and work. Some families like to have multiple kids close together, so they can get all of their kids out of preschool as soon as possible. Other families may find the prospect of multiple children in diapers to be horrifying, so they plan for longer spaces between the kids.

By all means make a plan, but in many families pregnancies do not occur precisely when expected. Having children is a great adventure, with many surprises. Don't make any plans that will disappoint you when they don't occur.

HOW CAN I GET MY KIDS TO STOP FIGHTING?

Review Chapter 24 for background information on the five essential components of discipline. Sibling fighting is a good example of how you can apply these principles.

Be clear about the rules. You can insist on no physical fighting, and no name calling, but you can't enforce a rule that kids aren't allowed to disagree. (In fact, siblings settling problems on their own is good practice for later.)

Use positive reinforcement. When siblings are playing nicely, most parents are eager to use that time to do their own things: read the mail, go to the bathroom, spend some quiet time enjoying a hobby. But if you ignore your children when they're good, they're more likely to stop being good just to get your attention. Next time your children are sharing something or making up a game together, take a moment for some positive reinforcement.

- *Good*: "Thanks guys!"
- *Better*: "I like the way you're playing together. You are making me proud!"
- *Best*: "Wow, you made up a neat game! I'm going to leave this plate with two cookies here for when you're done!"

Use appropriate punishments. If you hear your children physically fighting or using abusive language, immediately and without further questions or comments put them in separate rooms. Leave them alone for five to thirty minutes depending on their ages, keeping both of them in time-out for the same amount of time. When you let them out, remind them with a sunny smile: "No fighting." You don't need to say anything else, and you should not try to figure out who started what. You'll never determine exactly what happened, and the questioning will distract from the important message that physical fighting is never tolerated.

Another effective punishment involves putting a toy in time-out. If your children are bickering over a certain toy, put it away on a high shelf where it can be seen. You don't have to explain why. Later, try to catch them being good so you can give it back.

Sometimes, older siblings become upset when their little sister won't let them play alone with a new toy. You can have a rule in your house: children are allowed to take a toy to their bedroom and shut the door. But don't go with them; stay in the living room to play with the younger sibling with a different toy. Most kids will only stay alone in their rooms for a little while before coming back out to join the family.

How Can I Best Prepare My Child for a New Baby?

Well before baby #2 (or higher) is born, start talking about baby things. Talk about where the baby will sleep, what noises a baby makes, and who will be doing what sort of new jobs. Buy a new baby doll so your older child can practice holding and playing. Some hospitals even sponsor sibling-preparation classes, which are nice for children who like school and will be proud of their graduation certificate. Stress that your older child can be a great helper, and that soon enough she can start teaching the baby all sorts of great things. Review the section on "magic time" in Chapter 24 for one method of making sure your older child doesn't feel left out during the busy time of preparing for and bringing home a new baby.

If your child is less than two, don't try to get her out of the crib before the baby is born. She's probably a decent sleeper, and safe and secure in her crib. You do not need her wandering around at night once the baby is home! Worse, many kids at least temporarily lose their good sleeping skills when they move to a big bed. If your child is at an age where crib sleeping is becoming unsafe (that is, she can climb out), make the transition to a big bed several months *before* baby comes home. Try not to make any other unnecessary changes at the same time the baby arrives. This is not a good time to begin preschool or insist that your older child start riding a bus.

Help make the arrival of a new baby fun by having wrapped presents that your older child can exchange with the baby. When visitors come over, they should first come to see the "new big sister" to congratulate her on a job well done. Visitors can ask the older sibling to show them the new baby. "Can you show me her toes? Wow, thanks for your help!" You can even have a few wrapped presents hidden away for visitors to give to the big sister if they forgot to bring one. Believe me, the baby doesn't care if he gets any attention, but the big sister sure does!

Now That I Have Two Kids, How Can I Always Be Fair?

You can't. Don't try.

It isn't important to be fair; it's important to try to take care of each child, addressing their needs individually. One child might thrive on lots of personal cuddles; one child might be more independent. Don't count the cuddles to try to even them out. Another example: one child might need a new jacket, and the other might say "I want a new jacket, too!" The best response to this is "Your jacket fits fine and is in good shape. You don't need one now."

Fairness is an important virtue. Encourage your children to think about being fair when sharing toys or when giving presents. Model good, fair decision making when it's appropriate and practical. But don't consider fairness a straightjacket. Parents cannot be fair all the time, and trying to be perfectly fair leads to bickering and arguing over details. It's better to try to do the right thing than to always be fair.

28

SLEEP, JUNIOR, SLEEP

Though we have no idea why people need sleep, we do know it is essential for good health. Parents and their children need adequate, good-quality sleep to stay healthy, alert, and agreeable. Still, many preschoolers fight sleep. They yell at bedtime, they scream at night, and they sneak out of their beds when they know their parents are too exhausted to send them back. It may take some coaxing and consistency, but most children can be taught to be great sleepers. Once kids sleep well they're more happy and contented—and so are their parents.

There is no single correct way to get the best sleep for your family. Some parents enjoy having their children share their bed. As long as they're doing this safely, neither grandparents nor pediatricians should object. In this chapter, I'm going to focus on creating a system of consistent *independent* sleeping for preschoolers. In my experience and in surveys of families, a household with children sleeping in their own beds works best for most families. However, if you've found that sharing your bed as a family works well for everyone—both the adults and the children—then you may not need to encourage independent sleep habits.

Safe Bed Sharing

A safe family bed should not have overly fluffy bedding, should never be a waterbed, and should not include gaps that can entrap a child. Parents must never consume drugs or alcohol that deepen sleep. There is also evidence that it is not safe for overweight parents or parents with obstructive sleep apnea to share a bed with their children. Because it is difficult to ensure that a shared bed is as safe as a crib, the American Academy of Pediatrics has recommended babies not share their parents' bed.

GOOD SLEEP DEFINED: WHAT CAN YOU EXPECT?

Sleep needs vary from person to person, and there are broad ranges of normal for different ages. Recent research has shown that young children probably need less sleep than had been recommended in the past.

- There is a large range of normal sleep at **every** age. No one can predict with certainty exactly how much sleep your individual children need.
- Newborns need on average sixteen to seventeen hours of sleep, though some newborns will sleep twenty hours or more a day. Newborns sleep a lot, but their sleep needs change quickly.
- Between two weeks and two years, babies need about thirteen to fifteen hours of sleep. Though children within this age range sleep about the same number of hours per day, they take fewer and longer naps as they get older.
- From three to nine years of age, about nine to eleven hours of sleep is sufficient.
- By age ten and up, nine hours or less is fine. Teenagers may have increased sleep needs during periods of rapid growth.

For children, good sleep means they're getting enough quality sleep without interfering with the sleep of the rest of the household. By age six months, almost all babies can sleep through the night. Many babies will do this even younger with some gentle persuasion. Babies should be encouraged by four to six months to go to bed earlier than their parents, so mom and dad can have their own time together. Happy and healthy children need well-rested parents who have time for their own relationship. This should be one of the goals of sleep training.

In the next section we'll cover how to gently train good independent sleep habits starting from birth. These guidelines are for healthy, term babies. If your baby was born more than a month early or has special health problems, you should discuss adjusting your sleep training schedule and expectations with your pediatrician.

NEWBORN SLEEP HABITS: IT'S NEVER TOO EARLY

Sleep training begins as soon as your newborn arrives. Demonstrate the difference between night and day by exaggerating the day's natural rhythm:

- During the day, all feedings should take place as soon as a baby wakes, and should be accompanied by talking and activity. After meals, if your baby is awake take some time to talk and sing. You should try to enforce this pattern: sleep, then eat, then play, then go back to sleep. Don't be worried if this doesn't work every time—newborns will sleep when they want, and sometimes don't follow your plan—but try to encourage this pattern during the day.
- At night, there should be no talking, no singing, and little activity. Feed your baby in the calmest manner possible, and put your baby back down to sleep

after burping. The night pattern ideally will look like this: sleep, then eat, then sleep some more.

Again, these are idealized patterns. Don't worry if they don't always work; just try them and gently work to encourage your baby to follow your lead. If your newborn is especially fussy and can't settle, review Chapter 19 for tips on how to make it through this difficult time.

Two Months Old, Ready to Mold

By two months of age your baby will know night from day, and should be sleeping longer stretches at night. Now is the time to start to encourage your baby to establish the single key to a good night's sleep for the entire family: independent sleep associations.

Sleep associations are things in our surroundings that accompany us as we fall asleep. People fall asleep quicker and sleep more soundly if their usual associations are present all night. For adults, sleep associations might include a dark, quiet room; a comfortable blanket; and a nearby spouse. For babies, good associations are a white noise machine, a nightlight, and a thin special blanket. If any associations disappear later at night, you or your baby will wake and wonder what happened. That is why most of us wake up if a spouse sneaks out to the kitchen for midnight ice cream.

> ☞ **For a solid night's sleep, sleep associations must remain present all night.**

The single most important predictor of whether children will sleep through the night is how they fall asleep in the first place. If they fall asleep alone— that is, not depending on a parent as a sleep association—they will soon sleep independently through the night. Children who fall asleep with a parent are unlikely to sleep through the night until they are several years old.

By two months of age, babies are ready to start working on developing independent sleep associations. At this age, you should at least sometimes put your baby down awake. If there's a lot of screaming, pick him up for consoling, but don't give up quickly on the plan to put him down awake sometimes. Try again later. If you don't try at least *sometimes*, it will never work. It doesn't

> ☞ **The two-month rule: *sometimes* put your baby down awake.**

have to be *always*—if two-month-old Baby Joey is already fast asleep, just put him down. Next time, try to get him down a little sooner, before he's fallen asleep.

Begin working on your overall sleep routine. It doesn't have to be elaborate, but should be a set routine of steps that will become a cue for your baby to understand that bedtime is approaching. You might include bathing, reading, prayer, singing, or all of these in your set bedtime routine. As babies get older, make this routine rigid and predictable, beginning and ending at the same time each night.

You've Reached Four Months, Don't Forget Lunch

By four months, you should be able to meet the "sometimes" rule above. Extend that rule just a bit to further reinforce independent sleep associations.

You might even have to oc-casionally wake your baby from a sound sleep at the breast in or-der to fulfill this rule. Do it, and don't apologize. You and your baby both deserve a better night's sleep!

> ☞ **The four-month rule: *usually* put your baby down awake.**

There's a second key factor coming into play at four months that you'll need to address. Babies know exactly how much food that they need each twenty-four hours to grow and thrive. Neither you nor your pediatrician can know exactly what that amount is, but we do know a few things about their needs:

- Babies need more calories as they go from newborn to toddler years.
- Babies don't care if they get their calories during the day or during the night.

Babies' growing stomachs allow them to go longer between feedings once they are four months old. You could use that time to make day feedings less frequent. But keep in mind that if four-month-olds aren't getting all of their calories during the day, they'll be happy to wake their parents at night to eat!

So how do you ensure your baby is getting all the food he needs during the daytime hours? First, feed him frequently. Every two hours isn't too of-ten, especially if your baby is awake and happy to take more. Second, begin introducing rice cereal, offered from a spoon, between four and six months to increase the daytime calorie intake.

At this time you'll also be getting a feel for your baby's own preferences for sleep. Experiment with warmer or cooler clothes, a brighter or dimmer nightlight, or an open or closed door. As you discover what seems to help, tailor your child's bedtime setting to what seems to work best for your individual child.

At Six Months They're Insistent, So Be More Consistent

By following only the rules above—that is, usually putting your baby down awake, and supplying enough calories during the daytime—most six-month-old babies will happily sleep alone through the night. Some babies, though, are more insistent, and will be more difficult to train. For these babies, you'll need to stand your ground and enforce very rigid sleeping rules. Keep in mind that babies that are difficult sleepers do not get easier as they get older. They get even more stubborn and more difficult. The time for a little tough love is now, because it will take much more struggling and tears to get this done later.

First, review your sleep plan. You should have a consistent sleep routine that begins and ends *at the same time each night*. Your baby should have a special blanket, nightlight, and white noise machine that can run all night. Bedrooms should be comfortable and lack things that move and create shadows that attract a baby's attention. If you use a music box or something like that to reinforce when baby is put in the crib, the song should last only a few minutes—not long enough to fall asleep, just long enough to act as a cue. And you must follow the six-month-old sleep association rule.

 The six-month rule: *always* put your baby down awake.

Some babies will protest your leaving the room. What can you do about the crying? The best short answer is: "stick to the plan." You can go in and check on your baby once in a while, but keep in mind that by doing this you might be unintentionally reinforcing the crying. Your baby might be thinking, "Wow, if I keep crying, Mom will keep coming back!" Instead, you want your baby to think: "Well here I am again. Alone, dark, quiet, my crib, my blanket. I've seen this before. I might as well go to sleep." Your goal is a better night's sleep for *everyone*. It will only get more difficult if you wait until your baby is older to encourage independent sleep.

SOME PROBLEMS AND SOLUTIONS FOR INFANTS AND CHILDREN

Teaching independent sleep associations is the most important key to getting a good night's sleep for your entire family. Inevitably, there are bumps in the road and setbacks in the plan.

Case 1: Delayed Training

Lauren is now eighteen months old. Her mom found it difficult to enforce strict independent sleep associations, especially because her husband traveled. The family developed a bedtime ritual that ended with Lauren being rocked to sleep in mom's arms, then being tucked in her bed as mom sneaked away. But at eighteen months, mom is exhausted from waking three times a night to rock her daughter back to sleep.

In this case, Lauren's parents need to "reset" her sleep associations so that she doesn't depend on her mom's rocking. But it is nearly impossible to do this cold turkey. An eighteen-month-old can cry so intensely and for such a long time that few families would be able to stand it! I suggested that mom gradually reduce how intimately connected she was with her daughter at bedtime, progressing to the next step every few days:

1. Continue sitting with Lauren in the rocking chair, but only rock every ten seconds. You may keep Lauren facing you in a tight hug.
2. Sit with Lauren in the rocking chair, but don't rock at all.
3. Sit with Lauren in the rocking chair, but with Lauren facing away from you, your arms tightly around her.
4. Begin to loosen the hug step by step, eventually just loosely hanging your arms over her.
5. Move the rocking chair right against the crib, doing everything else the same.
6. Now Mom remains in the rocking chair, but Lauren lies in her crib. Mom can hold her daughter and gently rock her.
7. Gradually become less touchy, step by step; try holding with only one arm rather than two at first, and eventually just sit next to Lauren without touching at all.
8. Try not to look at Lauren, just sit next to her crib; gradually move the chair further away night by night.

The exact steps don't matter, but the goal is to gradually make a less intimate connection, night by night, in a way that Lauren won't protest. During this phase of training, if Lauren wakes at night, Mom should resume whatever she was doing at bedtime that cued her daughter to sleep. This process takes time and may require painstakingly small steps, but it will work for any child who is dependent on a parent to fall asleep. It should be adjusted to become quicker or slower depending on how stubborn your child is about learning nighttime independence.

In this case, it took Lauren's parents two weeks to get to step 7; from there, Lauren's night routine was independent enough that she stopped waking at night.

Case 2: The Curtain Call

Jared is four years old, and had been a consistently independent sleeper. Lately, though, he keeps popping up for one thing after another at bedtime. First he wants another story, then a drink of water, then a trip to the bathroom. These "just one more things" can drag out for almost an hour.

This is an example of a habit that can get worse with reinforcement—that is, as Jared learned he could get a little nugget of extra attention, he started asking for more. And because of this, his parents have lost their quiet evenings together. For Jared's parents I suggested a variation of what is called a "token economy." Jared is given three dimes at bedtime, and every time he pops out of his room it costs him one. After all three are spent, if he pops out again he is silently walked back into his room without any affection and guided into his bed. But if he uses fewer than his three dimes each night, he gets to keep the extra ones in his piggy bank to save up and spend on something he chooses.

This system had enough incentive and fun to work very well to quash those curtain calls for Jared and his family.

Case 3: The Ear Infection

Anna Claire had been a good sleeper until her first ear infection at six months. Now, it's two weeks later. Her pediatrician has rechecked her ears, and says she's fine. But she won't go to sleep on her own, and will no longer sleep through the night.

Good habits can be learned, and bad habits can quickly be learned to replace them. In this case, while Anna Claire was in pain her parents indulged her at bedtime with snuggles, and of course helped her at night when she awoke in pain. When children are ill their parents should do what it takes to help them feel better, even if that means straying from good sleep habits. Sometimes it can be difficult to reestablish a good habit once the medical problem has passed. Families might experience a similar breakdown in good sleep habits after a vacation.

To fix this problem, Anna Claire's parents returned exactly to the plan that was working before the crisis. They resumed the exact routine, ending with Anna Claire awake in her crib with her usual lovies and sleep associations. With confidence and consistency, within a few days Anna Claire was back to her good sleeping habits.

Don't worry about an older sibling who might be awakened by a baby's nighttime crying. For some reason, older siblings almost always sleep through the crying of the little ones. All of that racket rarely seems to rouse them.

Case 4: Programmed Wakening for a Bottle

Robert, ten months old, falls asleep alone without a fuss. But he always awakes at 2:00 AM for a four-ounce bottle. If his parents ignore him when he wakes, he screams until the entire building is awake!

This is an example of "programmed waking." Robert doesn't really need the four ounces of formula, but he's used to it. His parents fixed this problem with a sneaky trick. They quickly went to him when he woke, bringing a four-ounce bottle. But each night, they added more and more water to the bottle, gradually making the milk more dilute. After a few weeks, the night bottle was entirely water. Robert didn't find that bottle too satisfying, but never really noticed it was changing enough from night to night to complain. He started sleeping right through his usual 2:00 AM waking time.

If he kept on waking for the water bottle, I would have suggested his parents just leave a bottle of water in his crib at bedtime. He could take a few sips of that when he wanted to, leaving his parents peacefully asleep!

You cannot use this trick for younger babies, especially less than four months. Babies need to have their independent sleep rhythm established before you can "deprogram" an awakening habit. Besides, young infants should not routinely be given plain water, and babies less than four months might still need to eat at night.

Case 5: Davis the Sneak

Davis, who is four, falls asleep fine on his own. But he always wakes at about 3:00 AM and sneaks into his parents' bed. They don't even wake up, but find him in their bed each morning.

In this case I gently suggested to Davis's parents that they really don't have a problem at all. Davis falls asleep fine on his own, giving his parents the evening to themselves. His sneaking doesn't wake anyone but himself. I didn't suggest that these parents try to change Davis's habits.

Davis has a cousin named Meg. She's also four, and falls asleep on her own. But her parents are lighter sleepers, and her habitual sneaking into their bed wakes them every night. Worse, Meg is a restless sleeper, and once she arrives Dad can't get back to sleep.

This family has a problem that should be addressed. Any or all of these suggestions might work:

- Put a cot in the parent's room for Meg. She should be able to sneak in more quietly, without waking anyone. The parents can enforce a rule: if she wakes anyone, she is taken back to her room.
- Set up a reward system. Every morning Meg awakens in her own bed, she gets a sticker. Three stickers earn a trip for ice cream!
- When Meg arrives, one of her parents silently and without talking leads her back into her bed, tucks her in, and kisses her forehead. If this is done consistently and silently every single night, it will work—though it takes a while.

WHAT ABOUT MEDICINE?

There is almost never any reason to use medication to help solve sleep problems. Though Benadryl is usually safe, it does not in fact reduce awakenings or increase overall parental satisfaction with sleeping habits. Other medicines are stronger sedatives, and are not safe for even occasional use. Besides, no medication can ever get to the root of a problem to train better sleep habits.

In very rare circumstances, especially with a child who has developmental problems or when a family is truly in crisis, short-term use of a nighttime sedative can be appropriate. You'll need to discuss this with your pediatrician to understand the risks and benefits to make the best choice. In any case, medication for sleeping problems in children should always be viewed as a last resort.

THE SCARY SLEEP PROBLEMS: NIGHTMARES AND NIGHT TERRORS

Not scary as in serious, but scary as in frightening: nightmares frighten the child, and night terrors frighten the parents! These two night events can both be disruptive, but are very different in nature.

Nightmares are what parents still occasionally have. They're scary dreams that awaken the sleeper with a start. A person having a nightmare will at least for a little while be able to remember exactly what the nightmare was about. Although occasional nightmares will happen, some tips can reduce their frequency and intensity:

- Avoid foods with caffeine, including iced tea, colas, some citrus sodas, and chocolate. Some common medicines, including antihistamines, can also trigger nightmares.
- Avoid any video entertainment before bedtime. Even the calmest videos are very stimulating to certain parts of the brain.
- Avoid exposing your child to scary images and stories. This especially includes any television news.
- If your child has frequent nightmares, try to gently encourage a specific dream by discussing a happy scene right at bedtime.

Night terrors are entirely different. They are rarely seen in adults. During night terrors, children are not awake. Even if their eyes are open, they will not see their parents. They will not want to be held and consoled. Night terrors may involve yelling, thrashing, or even running. The next morning, children will have no memory of their frightening outburst.

Because night terrors often occur in clusters for several nights in a row at the same time, there is an easy cure for them. The night after your child has a night terror, wake her up about fifteen minutes before the time the event began. You don't have to wake the child fully—just a little nudge followed by a "go back to sleep" will be enough to disrupt the sleep rhythm, preventing a night terror from occurring.

Children who have night terrors are prone to having clusters of them again later, so you may have to repeat the process. Night terrors sometimes occur in the same kids as sleep walking, sleep talking, and teeth grinding. Talk to your pediatrician if these sorts of issues are becoming disruptive to your family.

Adequate sleep is required not only for good health, but also to keep family members happy and functioning. Children certainly benefit from a good night's sleep, and as a bonus their well-rested parents will be more relaxed and resilient. Furthermore, children who can fall asleep on their own will have parents who are able to have time for their own relationship. Though some children will become excellent sleepers without any training from their parents, most kids need at least some gentle encouragement to become independent. Though it's easier to train your child to be a good sleeper if you start early, it's never too late to work on developing better habits. The investment of energy and time to help your child become a good sleeper will help your entire family stay happy, healthy, and safe.

INDEX

About the Author

ROY BENAROCH, M.D., is Clinical Assistant Professor of Pediatrics at Emory University and a pediatrician with a private practice in Roswell, Georgia. The father of three children, "Dr. Roy" completed an undergraduate degree in Biomedical Engineering at Tulane University and completed medical school and his residency at Emory University.